# MANBOOB NATION

*An integrative medical model to low testosterone*

NATHAN GOODYEAR, MD

# ACKNOWLEDGMENT

I would like to thank all those that have supported me in the development and creation of this book. First, thank you to all those physicians that have lead the way in Wellness medicine. There are too many of you to thank personally here, but without your push for better health care, this paradigm shift may never have happened. Thank you to my brother. His expertise in writing and his knowledge has been a tremendous resource and encouragement. Thanks to my dad. His help in editing and encouragement have been invaluable. To my wife and family, thank you. Thanks to my wonderful children. They sacrificed time with me so that I could research and write this book. My greatest resource of encouragement and my partner in live is my beautiful bride. I thank you for all that you have done to support me. In the good times and the bad, your commitment to us has given me the courage to pursue and declare the truth. Ultimately, thank you to God and my Savior, without which none of this would be possible. You are the source of all Truth.

# FOREWORD

Fifteen years ago I discovered that most of what I was taught in medical school did not help patients become well.  It became obvious when I, a board certified Obstetrician/Gynecologist, realized that  with all my knowledge  I could not help my wife who was experiencing hormonal problems.  I lived with my wife seven days a week, but conversely saw my  patients for only about  fifteen minutes each year.  What seemed to pacify my patients at their yearly visits did not help my wife.

I was at a lost as to how to help my wife.  I began to seek out information that would later help both my wife and patients live healthier and fulfilling lives.   As I did, I came to the realization that pharmaceutical drugs could not help my wife and patients.  I found the key to my wife's problem in bio-identical hormone replacement and functional medicine.  These entities, which restore the body to optimum health, enhance the body's ability to function at its highest level.  They help the body to correct hormonal and nutritional imbalances while addressing the impact of our environment, diet, genetics and lifestyle on our health.  Functional medicine allows healthcare practitioners to intervene when there is dysfunction in the body long before a disease develops.

Armed with the victory of helping my wife and transforming my medical practice, I began to travel the speaker's circuit to educate other doctors about my newfound knowledge. It was at a medical conference that I was speaking at in San Antonio, Texas in 2006 that I met Nathan Goodyear M.D., who was in the audience. Because he was also an Obstetrician/ Gynecologist, I think he had a special interest in hearing what I had to say. By the end of that two-day seminar we had become friends. It has been years since we first met. I have witnessed first hand how Nathan's burning interest and commitment to help his patients transformed his life.

This book is evidence of his commitment to patient care and service as a physician. Dr. Goodyear does an excellent job of documenting how the U.S. healthcare system is predicated on managing sickness and not health and healing. Unfortunately, wellness is not the desired outcome when most of our the healthcare economy is based on sickness.

Dr. Goodyear's book clearly inspires doctors to think differently. He has taken the time and effort to write a book to educate other about obesity, metabolic syndrome and male hormone deficiencies. This book goes beyond what is usually discussed about these conditions. Dr. Goodyear focuses on utilizing bio-identical hormone replacement and functional medicine to eradicate these conditions that are at near epidemic levels.

I encourage you to open your mind and absorb what Dr. Goodyear has to share with you. This may be the best investment you can make towards improving your health.

Eldred Taylor, MD

# TABLE OF CONTENTS

# PREFACE

Men are not the men that their grandfathers were. Obesity is on the increase. Estrogen production in men is on the incline. Testosterone and sperm count are on the decline.

What is the physiologic impact on the health of men?

Better yet, what is the cause.

To know the physiologic impact, one must know the underlying cause. Is low Testosterone the problem. Or, is low Testosterone merely the effect of the cause? The effect that produces the symptoms and physical signs are the result of low T, but should that be the focus?

In fact, the low Testosterone epidemic is not the cause, but is simply the effect. So what is the cause?

Marketing would have us believe that it is all about the T. Physicians are not immune to this trap. Instead of "evidence-based" practitioners, we have become "marketing-based" practitioners. We providers practice medicine out of 30-60 second marketing bytes.

That is marketing. But what does the science say. Not, what do opinion statements say. Not, what do self-help books say. And definitely, not what marketing says. What does the science, bias and opinions removed, say.

There are 8 primary causes of low Testosterone:

1)   natural decline
2)   stress
3)   estrogen
4)   obesity
5)   inflammation
6)   toxins
7)   medications
8)   HRT

As Functional medicine practitioners, the source of the problem is our focus. A healing strategy for health care requires a solution based therapeutic approach. That is the drive behind "Man Boob Nation", a functional medicine approach to low T.

# CHAPTER 1

# CONFESSIONS OF A RECOVERED FAT MAN

6 foot 1 inch, 190 lbs, and 15% body fat. Now, that doesn't sound like a fat man. Yes, the 15% could be lower. But, let's look at that in context. Many years ago, that would have been 6 foot 1 inch, 285 lbs and I hate too even guess what the body fat percentage was.

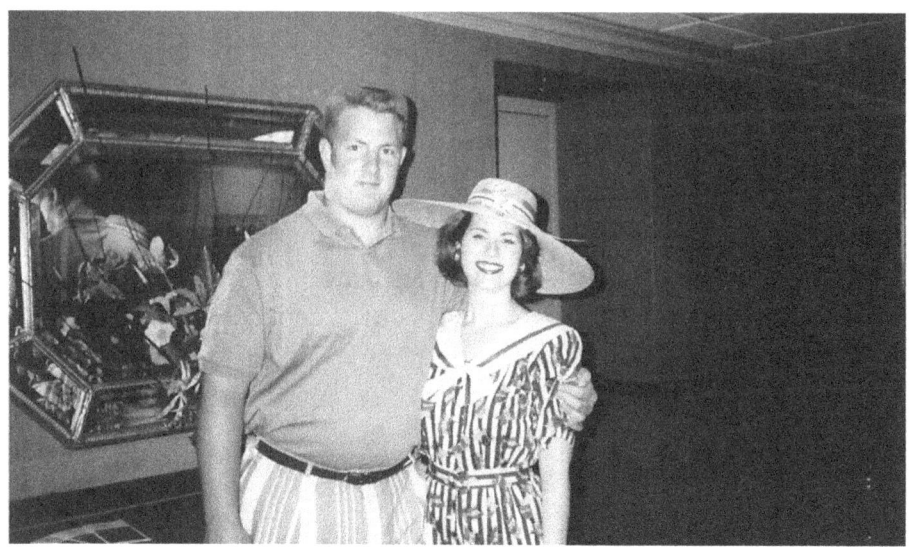

Yup, that was me when I was in college with my bride of now 22 years. Heck, that was me even into medical school and residency. I was 250 lbs even into my second year of residency.

That may not sound like a lot when thinking of a football player, so let me put that in to the context of clothes. My dress shirt size (neck) was 23 1/2, I wore a size 54 dress coat, and my pant size was a 46! Was I a football player with broad shoulders? Yes. But, I was fat!

Yes, I played college football many years ago. Now, I often ask people what position, they think that I played. It is great to get the answers. Wide receiver and quarterback are usually the most common answers I get. And the quarterback was close. I played center for 4 years at Louisiana Tech. Yes, I bench pressed 400 lbs and squatted 500 lbs. I can't remember the exact weights, but it was a heck of alot. The bench press and squat numbers continue to grow as do the years. As strong as I was, I was fat too.

Our diets were amazing. It is no wonder that the majority of linemen coming out of college are headed towards obesity. In fact, it is a problem that most football players will struggle with, given time. Just look at the retired players in the NFL today and compare them to their playing days. The quarterbacks and running backs start to look like the lineman and the lineman start to look like, well fat guys. It is rare to see exceptions to that rule.

The problem for these football players? They never adjust their lifestyles. As a football player–you are churning and burning. You may be taking in 10,000 calories a day or more, but you are burning every bit of that over the day of practice, training, lifting... When I was playing college football, my calorie intake was unreal. Just thinking of the food I use to eat makes me nauseated.

So, how much was it? What did it look like? I would eat 5 meals a day. Of course, there was the normal breakfast and lunch, for me and my size that is. Breakfast would be 4-5 pancakes, sausage, and bacon. How did my pancreas survive; I don't know. The evenings was where things got really crazy. Practice always started about 3 pm and finished about 5:30. Then, it was off to the dinning table. Think of the breakfast and double the size. Hey, I had just finished practice. Then it was back to the meeting room to review video of the practice. Following practice, it was off to subway for a footlong. And, I may even had some ice cream later, over my school work.

Then, there were the food orgies. I can remember a good friend of mine, now in the NFL hall of fame, eating a whole, family size bucket of chicken from KFC during film one evening. He ate a whole family of chickens! That wasn't a small, bite size bucket, but a family size bucket of chicken. My wonderful wife would make jumbalaya for all the starting offense lineman on monday nights and we would watch the monday night football game. That doesn't sound so bad, but she would make a recipe for 50 and 6 young men—would finish it off. That included sausage, shrimp, chicken, and rice. And don't forget the bread! Personally, when my wife and I would sit down for dinner, she would fix 12 tacos. She would eat 1 and I would finish the other 11 off.

Good grief, is right!

As I stated earlier, the weight pretty much stayed on until halfway through my residency. That was an additional 8 years. Some of the weight did come off as I dropped the number of meals from 5 to 3 per day. Some of it just had to. But, my activity levels dropped way off because my head was in the books and this led to a drastic decrease in my muscle mass.

There were no more 2 hour weight lifting sessions. There were no more off season stadium stairs. There were no more 3 hour practice sessions. I had changed part of my lifestyle, but I had not changed the other. I had decreased my calories in, but I had decreased further, my calories out.

I didn't know it yet, but my lifestyle was a set up for future potential disease implications.

Now, I am not a calorie in/calorie out guy. In fact, I believe too much emphasis is put on that simple phrase. My problem was the change in my percentages. I had turned my body's metabolic capacity on it's head. My muscle mass was on the decline and my fat mass was on the incline. How do I know? Pictures don't lie.

Yes, I had decreased my daily meals while significantly decreasing my exercise. However, my macronutrient (protein, carbs, and fats) remained unchanged. My percentage of carbohydrate intake had not changed. I had become a carb junkie during my football years. And it was beneficial, at the time. But now, that high carbohydrate intake had become a drug. A drug that was wrecking my metabolism. More on that later.

Sadly, two fellow lineman that I played with are dead due to cardiovascular events. One was due to a heart attack and the other was a ruptured aortic aneurysm. These good guys just didn't pass away recently. They died many years ago. One was in his late 20s and the other in his mid 30s.

Cause?

Metabolic Syndrome. Also know as MetS or Syndrome X. The name has changed over the years, but the underlying importance in health is the same. Metabolic syndrome is the doorway to disease.

In medicine today, when we cannot find the cause, we find a syndrome. A syndrome is a collection of items running together. In this case:

- Waist circumference > 40 inches
- Elevated triglycerides ≥ 150

- Reduced HDL < 40
- Elevated blood pressure ≥ 130/85
- Elevated fasting glucose ≥ 110

Individually, they don't say much. But collectively they speak loudly of impending disease.

How big is the problem? Approximately 25% of the worlds adult population suffers with metabolic syndrome[1]. Sadly, metabolic syndrome is not just an adult problem. Twelve percent of adolescents have been found to meet the criteria of metabolic syndrome[2]. A study of Canadian Qii Cree children, found metabolic syndrome at a rate of 18.6%[3]. Obesity is a major contributory to the development of metabolic syndrome. And according to the National Health and Nutrition Examination Survey, 17% of American children and adolescents are obese[4]. So, only expect the number of adults with metabolic syndrome to rise.

But, those statistics are in non-athletes with metabolic syndrome. Let's look at Athletes, because it is going to surprise you (maybe not). A study conducted on football players at "the" Ohio State University found, not only was metabolic syndrome a major problem, but it was predictive of future disease. No position was more effected than the offensive lineman. Their conclusion:

> "There is a strong association between obesity and both metabolic syndrome and insulin resistance in Division 1

---

1  Cameron AJ, Shaw JE, Zimmet PZ. The metabolic syndrome: prevalence in worldwide populations. *Endocrinol Metab Clin North Am* 2004: **33**: 351–376

2  Gungor N, Bacha F, Saad R, Janosky J, Arslanian SA. The metabolic syndrome in healthy children using in-vivo insulin sensitivity measurement (abstract). *Pediatr Res* 2004: **55**: 145A

3  Retnakaran R, Zinman B, Connelly PW, Harris SB, Hanley AJG. Nontraditional cardiovascular risk factors in pediatric metabolic syndrome. *J Pediatr* 2006: **148**: 176–182

4  According to the 2007-2008 NHANES (National Health and Nutrition Examination Survey)

collegiate football players. Lineman are at significant risk for metabolic syndrome and insulin resistance compared with other positions. This may be predictive of future health problems in Division 1 collegiate football players, especially lineman"[5]

Not only do the unsung heroes receive less recognition, they receive more of the negative future health problems. Sorry, just a little bias sneaking in.

But, that is the Big 10. Sorry, the SEC is just as bad. Reminds me of a conversation I heard on a sports talk show in Knoxville, TN. A caller called in to join in a discussion on college football recruits. His question was regarding a 6.6" 380 lb freshman in high school. The question? Is this kid healthy? What do you think?

It is ironic that this occurred on the best sports radio talk show in the country in Knoxville, TN. In 2010, a study of the Tennessee football team found a 46% metabolic syndrome rate among the lineman on the team[6]. This compared to 0% in the skilled position players. These are the young men considered to be very healthy by the average person. Yet, they have an increased cardiovascular disease risk due their metabolic syndrome. This is when they are at their peak physical activity. It has been my experience that this activity will only decline as time moves away from their football days. Unfortunately, the calorie intake and choice of calories does not change as well.

How does this compare to the general population? Sadly, not well. The general population doesn't fare much better. In fact, in many cases, the general public fares worse. According to the CDC data

---

5  Borchers JR et al. Metabolic Syndrome and insulin resistance in Division 1 collegiate football. Medical Science Sports Exercise. 2009 Dec;41(12):2105-10.
6  Dobrosielski DA Assessment of cardiovascular risk in collegiate football players and nonathletes. Journal of American College Health. 2010 Nov-Dec;59(3):224-7.

from 2011, 35.7% of adult American are obese. Thirteen states had obesity rates that exceeded 30%. Compare this to the year 2000, where no states had an obesity rate exceeding 30%.

What does the future hold? Always look to trends . The CDC recently published trends from 1960-2008 that showed a massive increase in obesity across the country (Figure 1) [7]. Trends show movement in numbers. One number or statistic, though terrible it may be, is itself static. But a trend of number shows movement in numbers. The obesity rate is only expected to increase. In fact, it is expected to reach 42% by 2030 [8]. Look to our children for the future. I use to live in Louisiana. Louisiana (2010 data) got a "D" grade from the Pennington Biomedical Research Center, on its Annual Report Card on Children's Health [9]. Why the "D" grade? Because, more than 47% of Louisiana children between the ages of 2 and 19 are obese and overweight [10]. The actual obesity rates for children 10-17 in Louisiana is 35.9% [11]. So, let's run with that number.

The health of Louisiana? Well, the Louisiana State Medical Board of Louisiana acts like Louisiana is #1. But, no such luck as a recent report ranked Louisiana as 50th in health. That is dead last! Unfortunately, the greatest obstacle to health in Louisiana are the policy makers, the Louisiana State Board of Medicine and the pol-

7  Ogden CL, Carroll MD. "Prevalence of overweight, obesity, and extreme obesity among adults: United States, trends 1960-1962 through 2007-2008." CDC. June 6 2011. web.

8  Finkelstein EA at al. Obesity and severe obesity forecasts through 2030. Am J Prev Med. Jun 2012;42(6):563-70.

9  "Annual Report Card on Children's Health...Louisiana Earns a "D" - Again." *Pennington Biomedical Research Center*. N.p., Sept 27 2010. Web.

10  Centers for Disease Control and Prevention. Trends in the prevalence of extreme obesity among US preschool-aged children living in low-income families, 1998-2010. JAMA. 2012;308(24):2563-2565.

11  Neergaard L. "Louisiana ranks in top 10 for adult, childhood obesity." *HoumaToday. com*. N.p., July 1 2009. Web.

iticians, and they should all know better. A growing unhealthy population will be a drain on the economy through healthcare costs and loss of productivity. That is a serious drain on the states resources and constrains any potential growth. But, of course a healthy population does not require their drugs, does not require their high dollar health insurance premiums and needs their doctor and medical provider less often. And yes, I am saying what you think I am saying. This financial burden will never change in their disease management paradigm, but can only change through a shift to wellness paradigm. Unfortunately, that is unlikely to change and Louisiana will always scrape the bottom of the barrel.

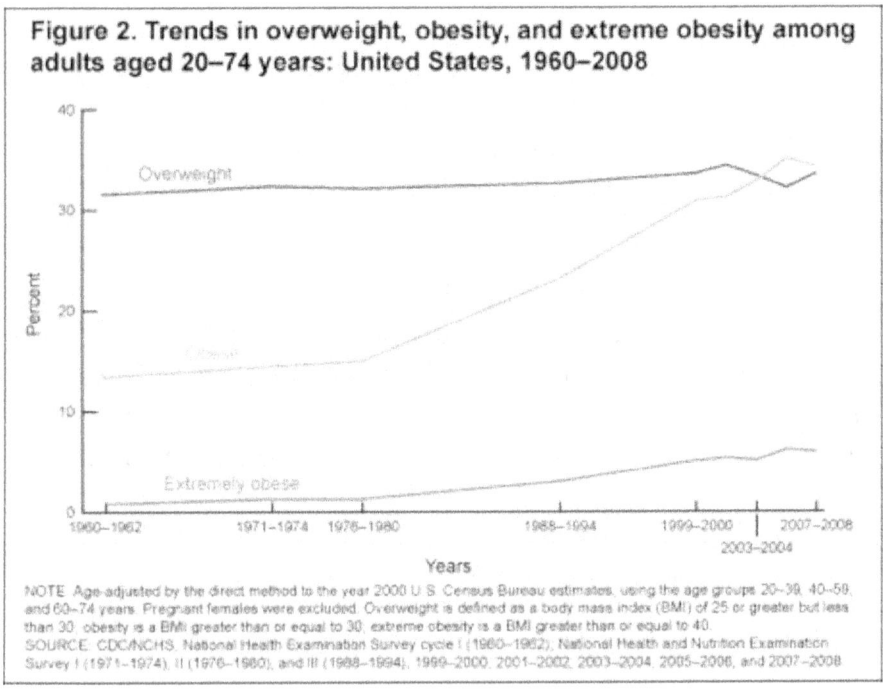

Figure 2. Trends in overweight, obesity, and extreme obesity among adults aged 20–74 years: United States, 1960–2008

*(Figure 1 Trends of obesity in America from 1960 to 2008)* [7]

Back to the 35.7% obesity rate in those 10 - 17. Let's say that the average life span of those children is 60. That is roughly 50 years of obesity and it's health related problems (that is the reason for the shorter life span). So, let's assume 42% of Louisiana adults will be obese by 2030, the population holds steady, and the costs stay stagnant (not likely). That is $2,665,622,736 annually. Now, multiple that times 50 years. The numbers add up really quick. Not only are they very, very big...they are unsustainable! And this is in a state that is trying to get it's financial house in order. It will never happen in the current environment. The leaders know this too. That is the worst part.

A recent report shows that the trend is expected to change for the worse. Instead of health improving, it showed that if current trends continue the obesity rate will approach 60% of the US population. That is obese, not overweight. Of course, the focus of concentration would be in the south with Mississippi and Louisiana leading the way as they currently do.

Everybody has heard the adage: "If it ain't broke, don't fix it". The problem is, in many states (particularly in Louisiana), health and the road to health is, in fact, broken. It is worse than broken. In Louisiana, there are deliberate obstructions to the health of its citizens.

I just quoted data above that showed the wrong path that Louisiana is on. My former US Representative, Rodney Alexander, told me at one time that he represented the 5th unhealthiest district in the US. Not something to be proud of. But it gets worse, the states and their associated governing bodies/associations are themselves a part of the problem. No place, is this more evident, than in Louisiana. Does that surprise anyone? The fact that Louisiana with it's colorful political history would continue to follow the path of "back door deals" is probably no surprise to anyone. Two recent online articles highlight the mind-blowing obstruction to health present in Louisiana. The very people elected and appointed to help their citizens are in fact, the very obstacle to their independence and health. The Alliance for Natural Health[12] and NaturalNews[13], have recently highlighted the obstructions present in access to "health" care in Louisiana. These obstructions are from the same regulatory agencies that were initially set up to protect the citizens of Louisiana. But, instead have, themselves, become the very problem that they were initially set up to prevent. How does the saying go, "absolute power corrupts absolutely". If you want evidence of that, just look to Louisiana.

This problem of corruption is no stranger to other states as well. The Texas state board of medicine is currently being sued for corruption in federal court.

But, they are not alone. They have willing accomplices in the health insurance industry. I know that many of you are shocked to hear that the health insurance industry has no apparent interest in your health; just your premium. They all have their part to play, but some are worse than others. Blue Cross Blue Shield (BCBS) is the absolute worst. In fact, it is quite evident that BCBS is actively trying to run integrative or functional medicine physicians out of practice. Do I have studies to support this? No, but observation, experience, and case law do just fine.

Case law? I know you are asking what this has to do with anything. It does, because it shows how health insurance companies go to great lengths to violate law to push profits, under the cloak of "Health". Basically, this is tantamount to a "shake down" of physicians across America. And seemingly physicians are glad to oblige.

---

12  "Louisiana State Medical Board Disgraces Itself (Plus an Update on Dr. Burzynski in Neighboring Texas)." *Alliance for Natural Health.* N.p., 14 Feb. 2012. Web.

13  Benson, Jonathan. "Louisiana State Medical Boards Continue Widespread Pattern of Abuse against CAM Practitioners" *NaturalNews.* N.p., 8 Apr. 2012. Web.

What insurance companies, like Blue Cross Blue Shield do, is they come in at a point and declare a treatment and/or test–experimental. Now, how do they come to this decision? They won't tell you. I and others have asked. They won't show a brief, they won't tell you the name or qualifications of their experts, they won't show you internal documents that support their decision, and they won't show you studies that support their decision. They will tell you that internal "experts" or experts that they have consulted with, have scoured the scientific data to make this decision. They then publish these decisions as "policy statements". But then, when you point out studies that contradict their own policies, they have no answers nor do they consider a change to their policies based on science.

But, I recently discovered that pharmaceutical companies employ people that consult with health insurance companies, particularly the medical directors, to help write policy for testing and treatments. You scratch my back, I'll scratch yours. At the expense of your health and mockery of the science.

They will then ask for repayment on the treatments/testing that were not deemed "experimental" at the time they were paid, but in retrospect have been deemed experimental. Let's think on this logic for a second. You eat dinner at a nice restaurant. Walk out satisfied and delighted. Then, sometime later, you decide that the appetizers were not gluten free as advertised and you find out the wine was only rated as an 84 by American Spectator. So you decide to send a letter to the restaurant demanding repayment for your dinner while providing little or no evidence to support your decision. Do you think you will get anywhere with that logic? Of course not. But, that is what BCBS does every day. A shake down on physicians. An obstructionist to health.

But, I said there is case law. And is there. I don't make claims without support. There is no right for BCBS to ask for any such repayment:

- <u>Great West Life Annuity Ins. Co. v. Knudsen</u>, 534 U.S. 204 (2002)
- <u>Sereboff v. Mid Atl. Med. Svcs, Inc.</u>, 547 U.S. 356 (2006)
- <u>Nicholls v. Prudential Ins. Co. of America</u>, 406 F.3d 98, 101 (2d. Cir. 2005)
- <u>Eastman Kodak Co. v. STWB, Inc.</u>, 452 F.3d 215, 223 (2d Cir. 2006)

And by the way, the first two cases were at the US supreme court.

But, it doesn't stop at the federal level. It even is at the state level. The Louisiana State Supreme court ruled the same in:

- <u>New Orleans and N.E.R. Co. v. Louisiana Construction Improvement Company</u>, 109 La. 13 (1902)
- <u>Bickham v. Washington Bank Trust Co.</u>, 515 So.2d 457, 460 (La.App. 1 Cir., 1987).

No opinion, just case law at both the state and federal levels.

Why do I point out the problems in health care? Sour grapes? Absolutely not! I think it is important that you understand that there are many obstacles between you and and your health. Many of those obstacles are disguised as "health companies" or are involved in "health care" and claim to be there for you. It seems counterintuitive. Why would they do such a thing? When you look at it from a business perspective, it does make some sense. It is a market decision. If you are healthy, then you have no need for a high priced premium to pay your medical bills. You would be just as happy to pay less for a high deductible, catastrophic plan and save your money over the long haul. And right–you would be. But for the insurance company that is lost revenue. And if you don't need them for coverage and doctors, they have no control over you. They cease to control you. You are free. Free to make your own health decisions.

So, with all these obstacles to health, what is the current state of health of Louisiana? Very poor. $1,967,483,000 poor! The current healthcare paradigm is not working to help the health of the citizens of Louisiana. Very few states actually do. The leaders are not providing leadership! Leaders are padding their collective pockets books at the expense of your health and wellness.

What do they say the definition of insanity is? "Doing the same thing over and over again and expecting different results" – Albert Einstein. And what does that make us that continue to follow in these leaders?

# CHAPTER 2

# THE COSTS OF NO HEALTH

"Health is like money, we never have a true idea of its value until we lose it"- Josh Billings

The rising costs of healthcare is a big topic today. And rightly so. In 2009, the costs of health care was $2.5 trillion. That is 17% of the United States GDP. In 2001, the cost of health care as a percentage of GDP was 14.1%. Percentage wise, that may not sound like much. But, from a money perspective that is an increase of roughly $1 trillion dollars in just under 10 years. This is the highest annual jump as percentage of GDP in history. And what about health insurance premiums? They are on the rise thanks to the increase in mandates through the Patient Protection and Affordable Care Act, better known as ObamaCare. Healthcare mandates account for up to 50% (see Figure 1) [14] of the costs of health insurance.

---

14   Terry, Ken. "By KEN TERRY / MONEYWATCH / February 4, 2010, 6:35 PM Health Spending Hits 17.3 Percent of GDP in Largest Annual Jump." *Cbsnews*. Cbsnews, 4 Feb. 2010. Web.

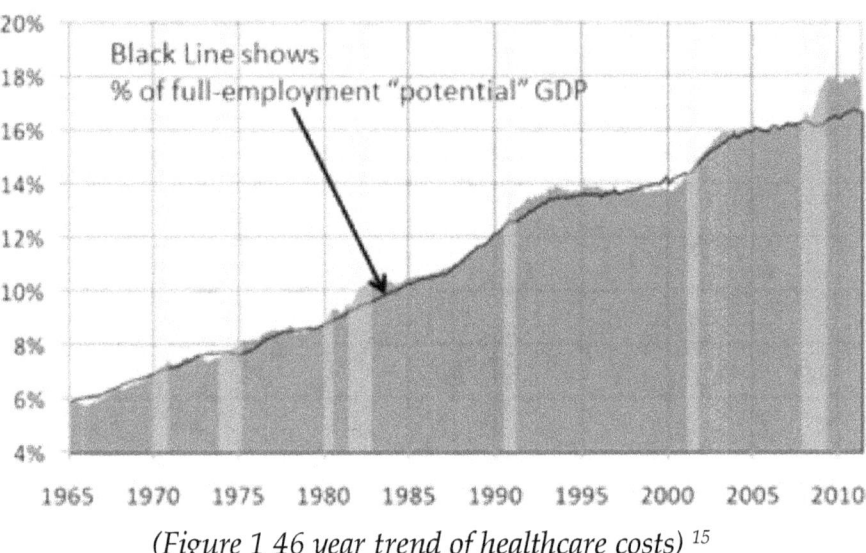

## Health Spending Share of GDP

Black Line shows
% of full-employment "potential" GDP

*(Figure 1 46 year trend of healthcare costs)* [15]

According to the Congressional Budget Office (CBO), the new federal mandates in the Patient Protection and Affordable Care Act will increase individual health insurance premiums by up to 30%. These premium increases are just an average across all the states. The change in premiums range from just a few with no projected increase (New York and Vermont), to the vast majority of states projected to have an increase above 50%. In Louisiana, the projected premium increase is 56%. States like Arizona, Arkansas, Georgia, Idaho, Indiana, Iowa, Kentucky, Ohio, Oklahoma, Tennessee, Wisconsin, and Wyoming can expect increases as much as 100% [16]. These numbers can only be expected to rise due to the yet to be written mandates of ObamaCare. In just one day in March 2013 (3 years after passage of ObamaCare), 828 new regulations were

15  Ward. "Telling a 46 year health care cost growth story in one graph. " *Reward Health Sciences.* N.p., Nov 12 2011.Web.

16  Senger, Alyene. "Obamacare: Projected Premium Increases by State." *The Foundry Conservative Policy News Blog from the Heritage Foundation.* Heritage.org, 18 Mar. 2013. Web.

published. That is 828 new regulations that will step in between the patient and his/her physician and become an obstacle to their health.

From a business perspective, what happens to the cost to the consumer with "middle-men"? The costs go up. Why do you think that everybody wants to buy through wholesalers? The middleman is removed and thus cost reduction. Look at how the healthcare costs have trended with the advent of the current insurance paradigm in medicine. The costs have sky-rocketed. But, this is the worse case of an administrative "middle-man"–the government.

What are we getting for these rising costs? Are we getting healthier? Are we seeing less Disease? Are we seeing less Cancer? Are we seeing less diagnosis of depression and anxiety? Are we seeing fewer prescriptions? The exact opposite is true. Unfortunately, the poor health of Americans is on the rise. In fact, the US consistently ranks low in quality and efficiency of healthcare and ranks #1 for the highest percentage of obesity at 30.6%[17].

When we talk about health, we are not talking about the cure of disease or about early detection. We are talking about outright prevention. This can only occur through a healthy lifestyle. This focus requires a paradigm change in medicine.

The current paradigm under which medicine operates is one of disease management. All the money that flows through this paradigm is under assault by the move of people who desire to be healthy. An improvement in health of the average US citizen is a threat to the established medical paradigm and a threat to their flow of money and thus their power.

The Picture of poor health is obesity and we are losing this battle. Obesity is the doorway to disease. According to the CDC, 67% of Americans are overweight, with 35.7% of those obese.

---

17  2005, OECD Health Data. "Obesity Statistics-Countries Compared." *NationMaster. com*. NationMaster, 2005. Web.

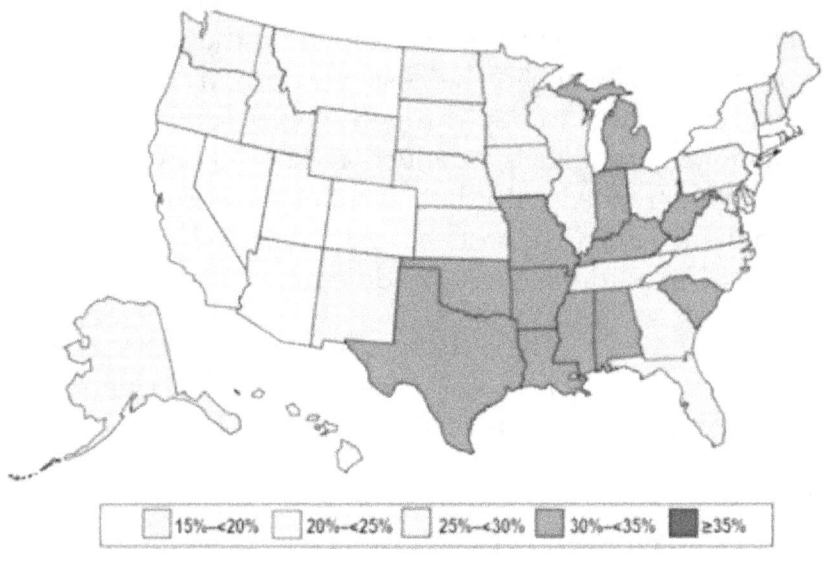

**Prevalence of Self-Reported Obesity Among U.S. Adults**
BRFSS, 2011

15%–<20%    20%–<25%    25%–<30%    30%–<35%    ≥35%

*(Figure 2 38 states with obesity rates 25%)* [5]

That is right, the number of obese adults in America have surpassed those that are simply overweight. In 2010, 38 states had obesity rates above 25% (Figure 2). Contrast that to 1991, where no state had obesity rates that exceeded 20%. What about the kids? Remember back to chapter 1, 10% of kids 2-5 are obese, 20% of kids age 6-11 are obese, and 18% of adolescents are obese.

So, what is the cost of no health? According to a study by the CDC and the Research Triangle Institute (RTI), the direct and indirect healthcare costs are as high as $147 billion annually [18]. Overweight individuals pay about 42% more in healthcare costs than comparable health individuals. This equates to an extra

---

18    CDC. "Study Estimates Medical Cost of Obesity may be as High as $147 Billion Annually." *Centers for Disease Control and Prevention.* Centers for Disease Control and Prevention, 27 July 2009. Web.

$1,429 out of your pocket annually. And this was in 2009. This has only increased.

What about individual costs? Remember, obesity is the doorway to disease. So, let's follow the path of disease development. The direct individual costs of obesity are $4,789 for women and $2,646 for men [19]. That is annual. Now, let's add in the disease progression costs for the individual, or the costs of the additional diseases that follow obesity.

First Diabetes. The diagnosis of Diabetes increases by 1 million annually. According to the ADA, the annual, individual costs of Diabetes is $11,744[20]. So, just the addition of diabetes adds $11,744 to the obesity costs. That comes to $16,533 for women and $14,390 for men respectively if obesity and diabetes are involved.

Second, cardiovascular disease. For our discussion purposes, this will include high blood pressure, Cardiac events, strokes, and associated treatments for an initial event. Costs for secondary events (ie second heart attack, stroke...) are excluded. Kaiser Permanente did a 7-year study of the direct, annually costs of cardiovascular disease. In this study, they found that the direct, individual costs of an initial cardiovascular event was $18,953[21]. A second event would increase the costs by 4.5 times. The costs just continue to add up.

What about Cancer? According to the ACS (American Cancer Society), the direct total costs were $93.2 billion in 2009[22]. For our discussion purpose, let's use prostate cancer (the highest incidence in men) and

---

19  "Individual Cost of Obesity Report." *Individual Cost of Obesity Report.* George Washington University Medical Center, 21 Sept. 2010. Web.

20  American Diabetes Association. Economic Costs of Diabetes in the U.S. in 2007. Diabetes Care. March 2008;31(3):596-615.

21  Nichols GA et al. Medical Care Costs among Patients with Established Cardiovascular Disease. Am J Manag Care. 2010;16(3):e86-e-93.

22  American Cancer Society. *Cancer Facts Figures 2009.* Atlanta: American Cancer Society/2009.

breast cancer (the highest incidence in women). For Prostate cancer, the average costs were divided into 2 categories: watchful waiting and treatment. The costs were followed over 2 years for 9,000 men. The direct individual costs of watchful waiting was $24,809. Compare this to the 2-year individual costs of $59,286 for the treatment group[23]. For post-menopausal women, the annual direct costs of breast cancer was found to be $13,925[24]. The costs of cancer are known to be a "U" curve. The highest costs concentrate in the initial phases and the last phases of disease treatment, with the lowest costs in the middle stages of disease treatment. Thus the "U" curve.

So, let's add this all together assuming a 5 year window of treatment and assuming aggressive treatment (no watchful waiting):

|                | Men      | Women    |
|----------------|----------|----------|
| Obesity        | $2,646   | $4,879   |
| Diabetes       | $11,744  | $11,744  |
| CardioVascular | $18,953  | $18,953  |
| Cancer         | $29,643  | $13,925  |
| Total (annual) | $62,986  | $49,501  |

Again, assuming a 5-year window of treatment. The total costs for men would be $314,930 and $247,505 for women.

23 Crawford ED, Black L, Eaddy M, Kruep EJ. A retrospective analysis illustrating the substantial clinical and economic burden of prostate cancer. Prostate Cancer Prostatic Dis. 2010 Jun;13(2):162-7.

24 Sasser AC, Rousculp MD, Birnbaum HG, Oster EF, Lufkin E, Mallet D. Economic burden of osteoporosis, breast cancer, and cardiovascular disease among postemenopausal women in an employed population. Womens Health Issues. 2005 May-Jun;15(3):97-108.

These costs include direct costs only. They do not include indirect costs. Additionally, these numbers are all pre-2011 dollars and are only calculated over 5 years. So, these costs are even higher today.

This disease cost hypothesis assumes the co-existence of Diabetes, Cardiovascular disease, and cancer simultaneously. Though the co-existence of all 4 diseases simultaneously is not common, it is very common for obese individuals to have diabetes and cardio-vascular disease simultaneously. Then give time, and the risk for the examples of prostate and breast cancer increase significantly. So, these costs may be spread out over a lifetime, but still would exist.

Then there is that thing called quality of life (QOL). QOL is some-thing that you can't put a $$ amount on. It is one thing to live to 95 or 100. But, it is another thing to live a high QOL to 95 or 100. The average American born life expectancy today is 78.48 years[25]. This has become very stagnant over the last 1-2 decades. Contrary to what many may think, this is one category that America is not #1 in.

So, how does one improve quality of life? The simplest way is to lose weight. We have already shown how obesity is out of control, how obesity is the precursor to many diseases, and how obesity directly increases health care costs. So it should be no surprise that studies show that just a 20 lb weight loss can provide signifi-cant health benefits for a decade of life[26]. So, if you weigh 200 lbs, you are just looking at a 10% weight loss. If you are at 300, where I see many men today, then your percentage weight loss needed is down to 6.7%. Now, who can't lose 10%?

---

25  Poladian, Charles. "Individual Cost of Obesity Report." *Individual Cost of Obesity Report*. N.p., 21 June 2012. Web.

26  "Modest Weight Loss can have Lasting Health Benefits, Research Shows." *Modest Weight Loss can have Lasting Health Benefits, Research Shows*. American Psychological Association, 2 Aug. 2012. Web.

As you can see, the health care cost problem is primarily one due to the increasing poor health of our citizens. If the people of America are healthy, their need and utilization of healthcare will decline.

Obviously, America is not getting healthier and the costs of healthcare are not going down. According to the Congressional Budget Office (CBO), the costs of healthcare will exceed that of discretionary spending by 2016[27]. The disease focus model is not working to improve the health of Americans. We need a disease model to treat disease when it exists. However, the disease model is not the approach for health and disease prevention. We need a new health and wellness model. This can only be accomplished through an individual, customized, metabolic approach.

And the future? What do trends show? Time will tell.

As Thomas Edison stated, "the doctor of the future will give no medicine but will interest his patients in the care of the human frame, in diet and in the cause and prevention of disease". Somehow I don't think Thomas Edison would take too kindly to what medicine today has become. Medicine today has made sickness a way of life. Medicine today is a band-aid paradigm with no focus on the cause of disease. This book will look at the low Testosterone problem in men today from a solutions-based approach provided through an integrative medical paradigm–the future of healthcare here and now.

---

27  McBride, William. "CBO: Federal Healthcare Spending will exceed Discretionary Spending by 2016." *Tax Foundation*. Congressional Budget Office, 31 Aug. 2012. Web.

# CHAPTER 3

# THE GROWING PROBLEM

No pun intended.

We all know the symptoms well. It is all over the TV, radio, and internet these days. Watching football with my kids these days has become a hazard. Especially with my girls. Monday night football has become an introduction into the "birds and the bees" discussion. Every other commercial is for ED. I understand this is a growing problem, but come on. There is dad, "what is a screen pass". Dad, "what is a penalty". Dad, "what is an erection lasting 4 hours?"–Really!

These commercials have a man sitting in a tub on the beach. Life is good, but why is his wife sitting in a separate tub on the beach. I never got that.

Marketing I guess. But it does not matter what marketing says, what matters is physiology. The body doesn't care what we think should happen, the body just does what it is designed to do.

Marketing does not match up with physiology. Marketing is about generating money and physiology is about generating health.

The growing problem? It is low Testosterone or more popularly known as "low T".

To define the problem. the medical field likes to come up with fancy names to categorize people into. Kind of like the government and it's commissions. And as in those instances, all words and no actions. Nothing is ever gets done. The problem is "managed", not corrected, and nothing is done to solve the problem. We have become a society of words rather than a society of actions. Ever heard, "you will know them by their actions"? That is a quote from the bible. It does not say you will know them by their words. In fact, it warns of the dangers of the tongue: "out of the mouth, the heart speaks".

So, what does the medical community call the problem? Testicular Dysgenesis Syndrome (TDS). What?! That is not a solution, it is just a name. Now that you know the name of the problem, you can fix it, right? Of course not and that is the problem. A name is just a name–a label. The name provides comfort, the name provides solutions. Or does it? The name does nothing in getting the patient to a solution to their problem. The name does nothing to provide the physician the ability to provide solution based therapies. The name does nothing to provide a pathway to health. We are no closer to fixing the problem, just providing a label and a band-aide. TDS is just lip service.

No solution is provided. We in medicine have a habit of putting what our patients tell us into fancy words that say the same thing. The perfect example is a person that comes in and says, "I hurt all over, my joints, my muscles..." Medicine's answer? You have fibromyalgia. What did we just do? We just told you in latin what you just told us. Now, the question is, does that get us anywhere? Does it provide a pathway to a core based solution? Of course, the answer is no.

The problem is in fact low Testosterone or Testicular Dysgenesis Syndrome, as defined by the traditional medical community. But the question is why. Let's look at it from a business perspective. Say your business is underwater. Profits are down and overhead is up. Then you are told you have "Profit Dysgenesis Syndrome". Can you imagine if you hired a consultant to evaluate your business and that is what they came back with? Of course that is ridiculous, but the appropriate analysis would then be why? Why have profits dropped and why has overhead increased? These are the correct. What is driving the problem(s). That is where the solution lies.

Let's look deeper at the numbers and discuss the causes later. The numbers problem can be found in both testosterone levels and in sperm quality.

Testosterone is on the decline, there is no questioning that. A very thorough study from the Journal of Clinical Endocrinology and Metabolism in 2004[28], showed that total testosterone levels have progressively declined in men.

---

28  Travison TG et al. A population-level decline in serum testosterone levels in American men. J Clin Endocrinol Metab. 2006 Oct 24.

# Testosterone levels have declined ~15% from 1987 to 2004

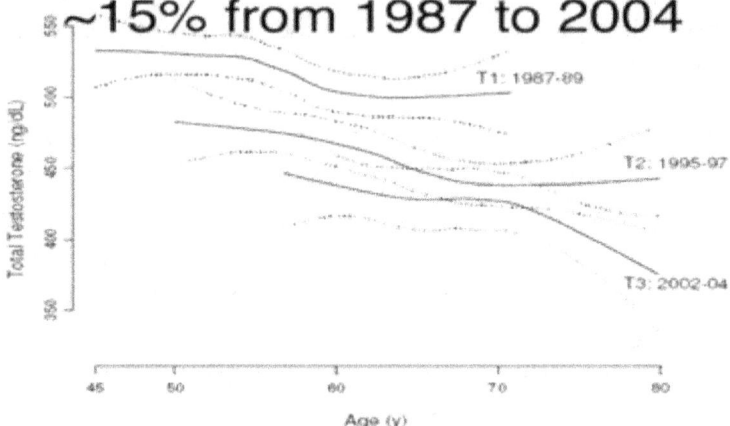

- <u>Travison TG</u> et al. A population-level decline in serum testosterone levels in American men. J Clin Endocrinol Metab. 2006 Oct 24

*(Figure 1 Testosterone levels on the decline)* [1]

The study followed the population levels of testosterone in men from 1987 to 2004 and found the levels of Testosterone were on the way down. These levels were not just declining in the elderly male population, but also in young men in their 30s and 40s as well. Worse, the trend seems to be increasing.

One flaw with this study. This study only showed levels as "Total Testosterone". This doesn't reflect tissue levels of testosterone. More on that later.

Another study[29] looked at the differences in the variation in testosterone levels in different populations. What they found, was that the greatest decline was in Americans less than 30. So, testosterone is not only decreasing in the elderly, but testosterone is on

---

29  Ellison PT et al. Population variation in age-related decline in male salivary testosterone. Hum Reprod. 2002;17(12):3251-3253.

the decline in men less than 30. Worse, the greatest decline, by age group, was found in men less than 30.

Still another study[30] found the total decline of testosterone in men at 47% over a life time. A recent study of 3,271 Finnish men were found to have progressive decline in serum testosterone levels when different cohorts (groups) were evaluated at 1972, 1977, and 2002[31].

If all that doesn't depress you, the following statistics regarding sperm quality will make the problem look even more bleak. One in 5 men between the ages of 18-25 have abnormal sperm counts. In 1940, the average male sperm count was 100 million sperm per ml. A 2010 Danish study[32] showed those levels had dropped to an average of 60 million per ml. That is a 50% decline in sperm count on average and 15 to 20% of young men have sperm counts less than 20 million. I guess our fathers and grandfathers were better men; or more accurately, we are half the men our grandfathers were. Throw in the 47% decline in testosterone levels through the life of a man and you glimpse the extent of the problem.

The conclusion? Men are dying half the men they were in their youth. The problem is that the average man in his youth is half the man his grandfather was at the same age.

With reference to declining sperm quality, the jury has been out, but recent publications are starting to provide clear indications that things are changing.

---

30  Morley JE et al. Validation of salivary testosterone as a screening test for male hypogonadism. The Aging Male. Sept 2006;9(3):165-169.

31  Perheentupa A et al. A Cohort Effect on Serum Testosterone levels in Finnish Men. Eur J Endocrinol. Nov 15, 2012.

32  "Out for the count: Why levels of sperm in men are falling". The Independent. April 26 2010.

A 2012 study published in the British Medical Journal [33] looked at sperm count, concentration, and morphology. They compared men in the general population today to men in infertile couples in the 1940s. What they found is that the sperm concentration and count is lower today than in the infertile couples in the 1940s. The only point at which sperm concentration and sperm count exceed that of the 1940s population are those with extremely low concentrations and counts. Additionally, they found an increase in abnormal sperm form, or morphology.

The debate on sperm morphology is really starting to close with the recent publication of the journal Human Reproduction [34]. This study evaluated 26,609 men between the ages of 18 and 70 over a 17 year retrospective study. The study looked at men in couples seeking their first assisted reproductive treatment. What they found is startling. This study found a 32% decline in sperm concentration over the 17 year study period. That was an annual 1.9% decline annually. Additionally, they found a 33.4% decrease in the mean percentage of normal sperm ie. the sperm had a 33.4% increase in abnormal form.

As you can see from the above studies, Infertility is no longer just a woman thing. Men, more and more are playing a significant role in infertility. In my residency, women were always considered to be the primary component in infertility. But now? Well, we just aren't the men that we use to be.

We have all heard of the frogs in the amazon that no longer seem to have an identifiable male species. We discount it as some weird, obscure story of some freakish frog thing in the amazon. Sorry

---

33  Jorgensen N et al. Human semen quality in the new millennium: a prospective cross-sectional population-based study of 4,867 men. BMJ.2012;2.

34  Rolland M, Moal J Le, Wagner V, Royere D, Mouzon J De. Decline in semen concentration and morphology in a sample of 26 609 men close to general population between 1989 and 2005 in France. Human Reproduction. published online Dec 4, 2012.

guys, but those frogs are us, and that amazon is these United States! And now, as the French study shows, the problem is spreading.

According to the marketing hype, low Testosterone is all about symptoms. We are all familiar with the heavily marketed:

- decreased libido
- erectile dysfunction
- loss of strength
- loss of muscle mass

But are you familiar with the less known symptoms due to low T?

- fatigue
- anemia
- depressed mood
- irritability
- loss of initiative
- loss of goals
- decreased cognitive function
- loss of motivation

And last listed: gynecomastia or MAN BOOBS.

But, low Testosterone is not just about symptoms. It is also about disease. Low T has been linked to the following pre-disease and disease states in men:

- inflammation
- insulin resistance
- Diabetes
- Metabolic Syndrome
- Atherosclerosis

- elevated cholesterol
- Hypertension

So, you could say that low T is associated with increased mortality. And that statement would be true. Studies have clearly shown an association between low testosterone and increased mortality due to cardiovascular disease (CVD) [35] [36]. Low testosterone is not just exclusive to mortality due to CVD. Low Testosterone is associated with an increase in all cause mortality rate in men. All-Cause! A meta-analysis of 820 studies published in the Journal of Clinical Endocrinology and Metabolism[37] in 2011 concluded: "low endogenous testosterone levels are associated with increased risk of all-cause and CVD death". These are not publications from "throw-away" journals. These are publications from leading medical journals.

We all talk about low T or low Testosterone. But what is low T by the numbers? What is a normal testosterone level. What is the best way to evaluate testosterone?

First, we don't make a lot of testosterone. We only make about 5-10 mg of testosterone daily. Not much, huh. Kind of makes you question the high dosages used in male testosterone replacement today. Because that 5-10 mg of daily testosterone production occurs at 20 to 22 [38]. If we only needed 10 mg of testosterone daily at an age when we were chasing everything with a skirt, why do we need testosterone at 30 to 60 mg when we are in our 40s and 50s?

35 Giovanni C et al. Hypogonadism as a risk factor for cardiovascular mortality in men: a meta-analytic study. European Journal of Endocrinology. 2011;165:687-701.

36 Malkin CJ et al. Low serum testosterone and increased mortality in men with coronary heart disease. Heart. 2010;96:1821-1825.

37 Araujo AB et al. Clinical Review: Endogenous Testosterone and Mortality in Men: A systematic Review and Meta-analysis. Journal of Clinical Endocrinology and Metabolism. Aug 3, 2011.

38 Whitehead NS. Endocrinology: An Integrated Approach. Oxford: BIOS Scientific Publishers;2001.

Reminds me of a 67 year old man that presented to me with severe fatigue. As I was taking his history, he caught my attention when he mention "his nephrologist". He didn't have any kidney diseases listed in his past medical history. I inquired about the reason for his nephrologist. He was seeing the nephrologist for frequent phlebotomies. He was having to give blood every 3-4 weeks due to a condition called polycythemia. This is a known side effect of too much testosterone replacement. He was on testosterone injections weekly, testosterone pellets every 4 months and human chorionic gonadotropin (HCG) injections to raise endogenous testosterone levels. This man was being massively overdosed with testosterone. He literally was drowning in a pool of testosterone. Guys, as I stated in the paragraph above, if we didn't need to give blood due to excessive testosterone when we were 20 and chasing everything with a skirt, then we sure don't need to give blood when we are 50 or 60 and on testosterone therapy. More is not always better.

I referenced the study earlier that showed a decline in total Testosterone. Total testosterone does not reflect the active portion of testosterone. Total levels will include both bound and unbound testosterone. Testosterone is lipophillic, or fat loving. Blood is mainly water. Fat and water don't mix. Just cook and you will see that. But in the blood, testosterone is bound to proteins for transport. In that state, testosterone is inactive. And that bound testosterone doesn't necessarily equate to the level of testosterone at tissue levels. We don't know where that testosterone is going: is it going to the tissue, leaving, or just along for the ride. We just don't know. It is like the analogy of the FedEx trucks. You can have 100 FedEx trucks drive by your house. But unless, one stops you don't get any delivery. And that is good picture of what we currently believe that testosterone in the blood is showing us. Just the FedEx trucks. We don't know if they are coming or going, or just out for a sunday drive.

What we need to look at is the active, or free testosterone. This is the unbound fraction (Wait, I thought you had said testosterone in the blood is bound). Your memory is correct. That is the reason that blood is a poor specimen of evaluation for testosterone: from a functional perspective. Treatment based on blood testosterone levels usually results in massive overdosing. Remember, we only made 5-10 mg daily in our early twenties. If we didn't need more than 10 mg daily when we men were chasing everything with a skirt, we sure don't need it in our 40s and 50s. Looking at testosterone levels through blood is like looking through the wrong window. The best window to evaluate testosterone is through saliva.

Saliva is the best specimen to evaluate lipophillic hormones like testosterone. Why? Because saliva is showing the active, free form of the hormones. The hormone level in saliva is equal to the hormone levels in the salivary cell [39] [40] [41]. Additionally, a hormone in blood is in transport. While in transport, the hormone is bound to transport proteins. This protein-hormone complex is inactive. It has been estimated that 95% or more of hormone is protein bound and inactive. This ranges from 95% for progesterone and 98% for testosterone. A recent study comparing saliva, blood, and urine for the diagnosis for Cushing's syndrome, concluded that saliva was the method of choice [42].

In contrast, the hormone inside the cell is free of the transport protein.

39  Groschl M. Current Status of Salivary Hormone Analysis. Clin Chemistry. Nov 2008;54(11):1759-1769.

40  Riad FD, Read GF, Walker RF, Griffiths K. Steroids in saliva for assessing endocrine function. Endocr Rev. 1982;3:367-395.

41  Vining RF, McGinley RA, Symons RG. Hormones in saliva: mode of entry and consequent implications for clinical interpretation. Clin Chem. 1983;29:1752-1756.

42  Sakiharra S et al. Evaluation of plasma, salivary, and urinary cortisol levels for diagnosis of Cushing's Syndrome. Endorine Journal. 2010;57(4):331-337.

A hormone is simply a message. A hormone is produced in one place, transported to another, to then go inside the cell to turn things off and on. So, why would you look at hormones in any place other than the sight of action. Beyond that, the receptors for these lipophillic hormones (sex hormones, stress hormones...) are mostly inside the cell. Again, no reason to look in the blood when the free hormones and the receptors are inside the cell.

To be fair, free testosterone can be calculated. Did you notice that? Calculated. There is a formula that uses total testosterone, sex hormone binding globulin (SHBG), and albumin to calculate free testosterone. This is a fairly labor intensive and costly process– called equilibrium dialysis[43] [44]. Above that, SHBG can be a hard to control variable in that equation[45]. There are many things that can increase SHBG: estrogen, thyroid hormone (t4, t3), and cortisol just to name a few. Likewise, many things can decrease SHBG: low thyroid hormone, high insulin, oral testosterone, and obesity. A recent publication from Endocrine Practice found SHBG and Albumin to both be quite variable in the equation [46]. So, if SHBG and albumin are quite variable, the serum calculated free testosterone is unreliable. But more than that, why depend on a calculation when you can simply look and find the free hormone levels inside the cell?

---

43  Swerdloff RS, Wang C. Free testosterone measurement by the analog displacement direct assay: old concerns and new evidence. Clinical Chemistry. 2007. March 2008;54(3):458-460.

44  DeVan ML, Bankson DD, Abadie JM. To what extent are free testosterone (FT) values reproducible between the two Washingtons, and can calculated FT be used in lieu of expensive direct measurements? Am J Clin Pathol. 2008;129:459-463.

45  Loukovaara M, Carson M, Adlercreutz H. Regulation of production and secretion of sex hormone-binding globulin in HepG2 cell cultures by hormones and growth factors. Jan 1, 1995;80(1):160-164.

46  Guay AT, Traish AM, Hislop-Chestnut DT, Doros G, Gawoski JM. Are there Variances of calculated free testosterone attributed to variations in Albumin and Sex Hormon-Binding Globulin concentrations in men? Endocr Pract. 2013 March-April 1;19(2):236-242.

There is another new promising medium to look at hormones–urine. Urinary evaluation of hormones will provide another piece to the hormone puzzle. Hormone metabolites are easily evaluated from the urine. Metabolites are the breakdown products of the hormones themselves. Androgen hormone metabolites 5-alpha DHT, 5-beta DHT, and particularly 5-alpha,3-alpha androstane-diol [47] [48] and epi-testosterone [49] have provided significant insight improvement in androgen hormone balance.

You may be confused. That is ok. A lot of physicians are confused. Reminds me of a conversation I had with a fellow physician over breakfast. He oversaw 4 clinics in his town. One was where he saw patients, and the other 3 were managed by nurse practitioners. But, he was their supervising physician. Between, the 4 clinics, this physician was responsible for 100 patient visits daily. We were discussing data and how to stay current in the science. He was asking how I found the time to read 3-5 journal articles daily. His response to the conversation was, "I haven't found the need to read a journal article in 25 years". No additional commentary needed.

There is research that supports this physicians statement. The Institute of Medicine consensus report from 2001 found that it takes 17 years for science to reach the clinical setting [50]. Stated another way, the average physician is practicing medicine 17 years behind the current scientific knowledge.

---

47  Horton R, Hawks D, Lobo R. 3-alpha, 17 beta-androstanediol glucuronide in Plasma, a Marker of Androgen action in Idiopathic Hirsutism. J Clin Invest. May 1982;69:1203-1206.

48  Lobo RA et al. Production of 3alpha-Androstanediol Glucuronide in Human Genital Skin. JCEM. Oct 1 1987;65(4):711-714.

49  Jakobsson J et al. Large Differences in Testosterone Excretion in Korean and Swedish men are strongly associated with a UDP-Glucuronosyl Transferase 2B17 Polymorphism. JCEM. Feb 1 2006;91(2):687-693.

50  Institute of Medicine of the National Academies. *Crossing the Quality Chasm: A New Health System for the 21st Century*. March 1, 2001.

Another saying of the popular marketing is: "get out of the shadows". As if all the men with low T are hiding in the shadows. As if the men walking by everyday and are invisible. As if Low T is the new Alfred Hitchcock thriller manuscript just found! Come on... I say a better marketing slogan is needed: "Come into the light!" Truth! Novel concept, I know. But, men and their families will be better for it.

You can stay in the shadows if you follow the presumptions of low T presented today in pop culture and marketing. But open your eyes to the light of low T and start the progress to health. I don't have to look into the shadows to find low T: low T is everywhere.

# CHAPTER 4

# CAUSES OF LOW T

Men, we are not the men our grandfathers were. No, that was not an insult. That is a fact. And a bold statement! Our Grandfathers were of the greatest generation. The generation that fought world war on 2 fronts and pushed the cause of freedom against tyranny across the globe.

And what does that have to do with low Testosterone in men?

In 1940, the average male sperm count was 100 million sperm per ml. Fast forward to a study from 2010 and that average level had dropped to about 60 million per ml.

Almost a 40% drop in 2 generations (see Figure 1)! But the numbers get worse. Fifteen to 20% of young men have sperm counts 20 million per ml. And this was found to correlate with an increase in testicular cancer, rise in male infertility, and undescended testis [1].

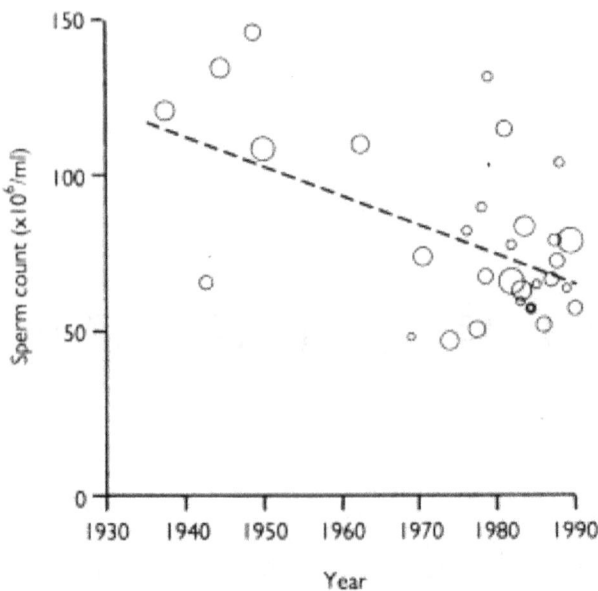

*(Figure 1 Decline in sperm concentration from 1930 to 1990)* [1]

That is all great, but what about testosterone levels? Because of course, that is what we are all interested in as men, right? The testosterone levels in men decline about 47% over a typical lifespan. So, we die half the men that we once were. But, that is just aging... right? A very telling study published in 2006 found that the testosterone levels as a whole were on the decline in men [51]. The levels were on the decline, not just in men in their 70s or 80s, but in men of all ages. Another study published in 2002 looked at the decline of testosterone in different countries [52]. This study aimed to determine if the low T problem was isolated to any particular country or region. They found that the greatest decline was in American men 30 years old. Ouch!!

---

51  Travison TG et al. A populatin-level decline in serum testosterone levels in American men. J Clin Endocrinol Metab. 2006 Oct 24.

52  Ellison PT et al. Population variation in age-related decline in male salivary testosteron. Hum Reprod. 2002;17(12):3251-3253.

We don't have the same testosterone levels our grandfathers had. We have half the sperm count our grandfathers had. We are, in fact, half the men our grandfathers were.

This problem, as I discussed in chapter 3, has been coined "testicular dysgenesis syndrome". That is what medicine does well today. The name should really be testicular disingenuous syndrome. The latest label given to the problem of low T is "male rejuvenation" [53] [54]. Both are a disingenuous attempt to solve the low T problem. The proper approach would be to forget the names and use the particular symptoms/physical signs to point the medical provider to the cause. Then a solution based therapy could be instituted that will minimize side effects. Remember that the 3rd leading cause of complications is physicians and the drugs and therapies (ie. surgeries) that we provide and recommend.

So, what then are the causes of low testosterone or "testicular dysgenesis syndrome" as it has been coined? What does the science say are the causes?

There are 8 primary causes of low testosterone.

1)    Natural decline
2)    Stress
3)    Estrogen
4)    Obesity
5)    Inflammation
6)    Toxins
7)    Medications
8)    Hormone Replacement Therapy (HRT)

---

53  Morley JE. Scientific overview of hormone treatment used for rejuvenation. Fertility and Sterility. June 2013;99(7):1807-1813.

54  Sigman M. Male rejuvenation: what the reproductive specialist needs to know. Fertility and Sterility. June 2013;99(7):1801-1802.

We will go through each one of them. Rarely, is it just one thing. Usually, it is a combination of causes and no two individuals will have the same unique combination of causes. Thus therapies will be individual as well. And, that is of course no surprise, as we are each "uniquely and wonderfully made".

That is one problem with healthcare today. For the purpose of "one-size-fits-all" approach, doctors and big pharma don't see patients as individuals, but almost as drones. People become dehumanized when they are referred to as patients, and not by their names. Socialism is alive and well in medicine today. So, let's look closer at the 8 primary causes of low testosterone.

## Natural Decline

First, is natural decline. Of course, aging is a part of life. It is reality. It is the reason I have the problem with the word "anti-aging". No matter how hard we try, we cannot stop aging. It is a fact of life, just as certain as the next sunrise and sunset. All we can do is help people age with a modicum of health and dignity.

As we have seen, the average man has a testosterone decline of 47% over his lifetime[55]. The peak testosterone production of a man occurs when he is 20-22. At the peak of our testosterone production, we men on average make 5-10 mg of testosterone daily. This is produced in 5 peak levels, with the largest occurring in the early morning. Compare this to the average starting dosage of testosterone therapy today. The average starting dosage, depending on the product prescribed, is 30-60 mg. I have seen many men have to donate blood due to a condition, polycythemia, that is the result of over zealous testosterone therapy. I have seen men with testosterone pellets, getting weekly testosterone injections, using daily testosterone gel. I

---

55 Morley JE et al. Validation of salivary testosterone as a screening test for male hypogonadism. The Aging Male. Sept 2006;9(3):165-169.

repeat, if men didn't need to donate blood when they were 20, then they sure don't need too when they are 40+ on testosterone therapy.

Sure, the guy with the pellet implants, injections, and daily gel feels great. His testosterone is at a place no mans should be. He is doping under the guides of a physician. Ask an athlete that is doping how he feels. He is of course going to tell you he feels great. I find the hypocrisy on doping crazy. Athletic agencies scour the earth trying to find their athletes that are doping. Yet, any man can go to his medical provider and get doped up under the guise of testosterone therapy for low T.

Testosterone levels do not remain stagnant beyond our 20s. Testosterone levels decline on average at a rate of 1.2% annually thereafter[56]. However, this decline accelerates to about 2-3% annually due to increased Estradiol/Estrone levels from increased aromatase activity. Any man you see with the "middle age bulge" or "beer belly" is showing off his estrogen producing factory. Where do you think "man boobs" come from? We will talk more about aromatase activity later.

But chew on this. If we start off at lower testosterone levels at 20 years old (as the studies show), then decline at an accelerated pace of 2-3% annually, you can see why we men have problems. Especially American men. Remember the study published in Human Reproduction from 2002? Testosterone decline is worse in American men less than 30[57]. This study compared declining salivary testosterone across different age groups in different culture populations. The conclusion better stated is: "the greatest percentage of decline in American men, when compared to historical averages, is in men less than 30 years of age". Not in men in their

---

56  Travison TG et al. A population-level decline in serum testosterone levels in American men. J Clin Endocrinol Metab. 2006 Oct 24.

57  Ellison PT et al. Population variation in age-related decline on male salivary testosterone. Hum Reprod. 2002;17(12):3251-3253.

50s or beyond. Less than 30. Such was the case of young 26 year old man I treated that couldn't achieve an erection. 26!

Is this accelerated testosterone decline normal? Is any testosterone decline normal? Sure some testosterone decline should be expected due to aging. Sure some testosterone decline is expected with aging. As a nationally known motivational speaker said, "I'm 73 and I have sex almost every night. Almost on Monday, almost on Tuesday..."

Aging is merely the accumulative effect of dysfunction. This dysfunction could definitely manifest itself in low Testosterone levels. But what is normal? This answer may elude us due to lack of historical data. There is limited data on natural decline in testosterone levels in the pre-obesity epidemic era. We Americans may just be seeing the new normal. But my contention is that this new normal is in fact not normal, but a result of the declining health of America.

## Stress

All those who are not stressed, please raise your hand. I often make this statement when I speak. Of course, I almost never see anyone raise their hand. And that is because we are a stressed out nation.

It has been estimated by the CDC that 90% of doctor related visits are due to stress. We often discuss stress as an unavoidable fact of life that's no big deals. Stress is very real. Stress is real physiology, and stress has real physiologic effects.

So what is stress? Stress is your fight or flight response. Stress is your survival mode. But, rarely are we in that actual fight or flight for survival. Even if we are, that stress response is short lived. Either you run away from the threat or fight it. And if you fight, either you overcome the treat, or the threat overcomes you. Either way, the threat resolves. Our problems today are primarily the result of chronic stress.

Analogy please.

My daughters love to watch animal shows. The zebra running from the lion in the Serengeti is the perfect example of the stress response in action. When the zebra catches wind of his predator, then the zebra's fight or flight response kicks in. The zebra must decide if it is going to fight or run. Either it turns and fights and becomes dinner or the zebra correctly decides to turn and run and get away. Either way the zebra's stress response is short lived.

Contrast this with the human stress response. As I stated above, we rarely see these life threatening events. But we have stress just the same. We deal with the "stressors of life". When I ask clients about stress, the response I often get is, "just life". Whether one deals with the stress of work, stress at home, or the often unrecognized physiologic stresses of (poor sleep, obesity, poor nutrition...) the response is the same. Our body doesn't know the difference. Our body doesn't know that there needs to be a differentiation between the types of stress. The body detects stress and it in turn responds. If this was short lived, we would see the effects that we find in the zebra analogy. But we live in stress every minute of everyday. So our stress response never turns off. It is this constant physiologic stress that causes major damage to our bodies.

So, what is the stress response?

The stress response is provided by the adrenal glands. The adrenal glands produce the stress response. They include norepinephrine, epinephrine, cortisol, and DHEA. The stimulus for the stress response comes from the brain. Particularly the pituitary and the hypothalamus. The Pituitary starts the process off with cortisol releasing hormone (CRH) and the pituitary follows up with adrenocorticotro-pin (ACTH) secretion. The result is adrenal gland stimulation.

The immediate stress response is provided through the production of catecholamines, epinephrine and norepinephrine. Also known as adrenaline and noradrenaline. These neurotransmitters provide the physiologic response necessary to meet the physiologic demand of stress in the acute term. You must have energy readily available to "fight or run". The commonly recognized symptoms: anxiety, heart palpitations, increased alertness are the result. Many would just describe this as an anxiety disorder. But in most of the time, it is just stress. Remember that 90% of doctor related visits are due to stress.

Cortisol and DHEA are the other major contributors and often the more recognized components to the stress response. When the body remains under stress, the body moves into a more aggressive, chronic stress response. This is with the above mentioned cortisol and DHEA. These two hormones continue the ongoing stress response and are associated with the majority of the stress symptoms and effects that we are all so familiar with.

But this is not about the stress response itself, but about the effect of stress on the male androgens. When in stress, we do what it takes to survive. Think about it. If you are running from the lion, will you need to stop and procreate? Of course not. The same applies to sleep, bowels... The body will put all functions not conducive to the flight or flight survival mode on the back burner and this includes testosterone production.

Stress is one of the primary causes of low testosterone. How? Adrenal cortical secretion of cortisol actually feeds back to the originating signals of testosterone production. Cortisol inhibits testosterone production through inhibition at the levels of both the pituitary and the hypothalamus. A double whammy of decreased testosterone signaling. The result is a decrease in leutenizing (LH) and follicular stimulating hormone (FSH) production. LH stimulates testosterone production and FSH stimulates sperm production. Thus you can see how an increase in stress and a corresponding decrease in LH and FSH production can result in what we see today: declining testosterone levels[58] and declining sperm counts and declining quality[59] [60] [61] of sperm in men.

## Estrogen

And then there was estrogen.

I recently took my family to a summer vacation to Disney World in August. We wanted to spend some time at the water parks. My 9 year old daughter commented that they needed to post a "no topless" sign at the beaches there at the water parks. And of course, I thought she was talking about some of the young ladies. But, she was really talking about all the men and their man boobs. It was at that moment that my eyes were opened. There were men everywhere in speedos with man boobs. Just imagine that for a picture.

Their problem? Estrogen!

Men don't make estrogen?! Oh yes they do. The scientific literature tells us we need to expand our thoughts on Testosterone. Testosterone is primarily the product of the testis. But it is not the end product.

58  Travison TG et al. A population-level decline in serum testosterone levels in American men. J Clin Endocrinol Metab. 2006 Oct 24.

59  Carlsen E, Giwercman A, Keiding N, Skakkebaek NE: Evidenc for decreasing quality of semen during past 50 years. BMJ 1992. 305(6854):609-613.

60  Auger J, Kunstmann JM, Czyglik F, Jouannet P. Decline in semen quality among fertile men in Paris during past 20 years. NEJM. 1995 Feb 2;332(5):281-5.

61  Dindyal S. The Sperm count has been decreasing steadily for many years in Western industialised countries: is there an endocrine basis for this disease? The Internet Journal of Urology. 2004 Vol 2 Num 1.

Testosterone is a prohormone. A prohormone is a hormone that has biological activity, but is then converted into other hormones. That primary male end-product androgen is dihydrotestosterone (DHT).

Have I lost anyone here?

Testosterone has biological activity, no doubt. But it is at a cross-roads. Either it is converted to DHT via 5-alpha reductase enzyme activity or it is converted to estradiol by aromatase enzyme activity. The bad news is only approximately 5% of testosterone is converted to DHT. The good news is DHT has 3 times the potency of testosterone[62]. On the other hand, Estradiol is the most potent estrogen. Pretty critical crossroads, huh. Either you take the road of manhood or you take the road of manboob hood.

What controls this balance is actually the balance of the 2 enzymes aromatase and 5-alpha reductase. We will focus on aromatase because we are focused on the estrogen effect on Testosterone. Again, aromatase is the enzyme that converts Testosterone to Estradiol. It also converts androstenedione (weak adrenal androgen) to estrone (still another estrogen).

So where does aromatase activity come from? Fat. Guess what is on the incline? Obesity. Studies tell us aromatase activity is present in all adipose tissue, but heavily concentrated in visceral and in subcutaneous fat [63]. That subcutaneous fat we are referring too is the expanding bulging waist-lines of Americans. Recent 2011 data from the CDC found that 35.7% of the US population was obese using the BMI data. Additionally, 13 states now have an obesity rate exceeding 30%. In the year 2000, there were no states with an obesity rate that exceeded 30%. Granted, the BMI is not the perfect measure. But the conclusion can safely be made that we, as a country, are getting fatter. Just look

---

62  Hemat RAS (2004). Principles of Orthomolecularism. Urotext. 426.

63  Blouin K et al. Pathways of adipose tissue androgen metabolism in women: depot diferences and modulation by adipogenesis. AJP-Endo. Feb 2009;296(2):E244-E255.

around you. Those men at the water park weren't showing off their war wounds, they were showing off their estrogen factories.

If we can limit aromatase activity in men, then we could safely assume we could reduce estrogen production. So, what increases aromatase activity in men?

- Age
- Stress
- Weight
- Inflammation
- Zinc deficiency
- Heavy alcohol use

Unfortunately, most of these can be lumped right in there with death and taxes. Age? sorry guys, no fountain of youth is on the way. There is no such thing as "anti-aging". We are going to age and with that age, increased aromatase activity. Stress? Would all those without stress please raise there hands. We are a stressed out nation, whether it is life stressors or physiologic stressors ie. obesity. Ever seen Wall-E? It is amazing to say that Pixar films have become the modern day Nostradamus. A recent Gallup-Healthways Well-Being Index found obesity on the increase in almost every age group from the 2008 to 2012[64]. And you have to throw inflammation into that mix as well. Fat is a hormone producing, inflammatory producing organ. So, if you are overweight or obese, you are inflamed. Zinc and heavy alcohol use are the only real causes that are avoidable or correctible.

Let's come full circle with this. As we age, we gain weight. That increased adipose tissue increases aromatase expression/activity.

---

64 Mendes E. In U.S., Obesity up in nearly all age groups since 2008. Gallup-Healthways Well-Being Index. Oct 24 2012.

Equally, the increasing adipose tissue increases inflammation signaling. The increased inflammation increases aromatase activity as well. The result is an increase in Testosterone/Androstenedione to Estradiol/Estrone production. OH, did I mention that estrogens increase inflammation in men? And remember that inflammation increases aromatase activity. Whew! Wait there is more. Additionally, inflammation causes disruption of insulin signaling and this results in insulin resistance. Insulin resistance results in increased adipose tissue. The result of all this chaotic metabolic dysfunction is low Testosterone. Which, oh by the way, increases inflammation in men.

The peripheral estrogen production from the bodies own endogenous testosterone will feedback to the hypothalamus and pituitary to decrease LH production and decrease testosterone stimulation. Estrogen also inhibits FSH production as well, which is a contributing cause for the low sperm count and quality.

## Obesity

I touched on obesity in the discussion of estrogen above. Obesity is on the rise in all age groups. According the the NHANES (National Health and Nutrition Examination Survey) 2009-2010 study, the obesity rate sits at 35.7% and the overweight and obese collectively sit at 68.8%[65]. The Extreme obesity rate sits at 6.3%. And according to the previously mentioned Gallup-Wellness statistics, these rates continue to increase.

But, what does the future hold? Look to our children to see the future. Seventeen percent of children 2-5 and 31.8% of school-age

---

65  Flegal KM, Carroll MD, Kit BK, Ogden CL. Prevalence of obesity and trends in the distrubution of body mass index among US adults, 199-2010. Journal of the American Medical Association. 2012;307(5):491-497.

children are either overweight or obese[66]. Well, that looks better than the adults, right? The answer is no. According to the CDC, the obesity rate for children aged 6-11 was 7% in 1980. So, the obesity rate has almost tripled in 3 decades. This is going to exponentially increase the obesity rate when they become adults.

Are all fats equal? Of course not. There is brown fat, white fat, subcutaneous fat, and visceral fat and they are not created equally. Brown fat and white fat are functionally different. Most think fat just is fat. However, fat is functional. Not only does fat play a role in metabolism, but fat can produce hormones and fat can produce inflammation. Brown fat is the "good" fat. Brown fat is involved in energy utilization. Brown fat is metabolically active. Brown fat burns energy to generate heat. Brown fat is actually good fat! Contrast that with white fat. White fat is metabolically inactive. White fat is involved in triglyceride storage. Guess which fat is dominant in obese adults? White fat.

The distribution of fat also reflects its risk. There is subcutaneous fat, visceral fat, gynecoid fat and more. Visceral fat is the fat that lines the internal abdominal/pelvic organs. Subcutaneous fat is that which is outside the abdomen/pelvis and constitutes the middle bulge. But the subcutaneous fat can also be anywhere. It can be concentrated in the abdomen, around the hips, the arms etc.

How does obesity contribute to low Testosterone? The visceral, but particularly the subcutaneous fat around the mid-section becomes an estrogen producing factory. In most men, the cause is not the fall in testosterone. The testosterone fall is really the effect. The cause is the rise in estrogen production. Remember from above, aromatase activity is highly expressed in fat tissue. So, as men gain that middle age bulge, high estrogen production

---

66   Ogden CL, Carroll MD, Kit BK, Flegal KM. Prevalence of obesity and trends in body mass index among US children and adolescents, 199-2010. 2012;307(5):483-490.

is the effect. The elevated estradiol/estrone levels feed back to inhibit LH production in the pituitary. The effect is to decrease the testicular testosterone production [67] [68] [69]. In many men today, because of the excess weight they are carrying, low testosterone is inevitable. And remember, with low T, all-cause mortality will increase.

A recent research publication summarized this relationship perfectly. The study looked at boys and young men between the ages of 14 and 20. They compared those that were obese to those with normal weight using BMI measurements. They found that those that were obese had up to a 50% lower testosterone level when compared to their normal weight counterparts[70]. Remember that peak testosterone production occurs at age 20. So, with levels 50% below average at 20, a future of obesity, low T and associated diseases may be virtually guaranteed.

## Inflammation

Like stress, inflammation in not an enigma. It is reality. Everyone is familiar with the cardinal symptoms of inflammation. Just recall your last injury. Whether the injury was a broken bone or a paper cut, the symptoms were the same (though the severity may have been quite different). What were the symptoms? Pain, swelling, redness, and heat. This is inflammation as it is suppose to be. Inflammation is suppose to be short-lived to provide protection against secondary invasion and to start the healing process. Once

67  Smet MD, Lapauw B, Backer TD, Ruige J. Short-term changes in serum sex steroid levels and cardiac function in healthy young men.

68  Kelly DM, Jones TH. Testosterone: a metabolic hormone in health and disease. J Endocrinol. June 1 2013;217:R25-R45.

69  Kang HY. Beyond the male sex hormone: deciphering the metabolic and vascular actions of testosterone. J Endocrinol. June 1 2013;217:C1-C3.

70  Mogri M et al. Testosterone concentrations in young pubertal and post-pubertal obese males. Clinical Endocrinology. 2012.

these goals are achieved, then the inflammation resolves as healing takes over.

The inflammation we are talking about here is the same; yet different. This is the same inflammation but it tends to be more low grade and it does not resolve. This chronic low-grade inflammation is able to subvert the normal regulatory mechanisms and thus what was intended to be short-term for healing purposes, becomes long-term with destructive results. The process of healing never can occur in the presence of chronic inflammation.

Let's get a better working knowledge of inflammation. Think of Inflammation as the language of communication of the immune system. For our purposes, we will discuss 2 components of the immune system. They are the Th1 and the Th2 systems. There is also Th3 and Th17 systems, as well as I am sure many yet to be discovered areas. The Th1 system is the cell-mediated immune system. The Th1 system is non-specific and non-direct. Think of it as your body doing hand to hand combat against invaders. No specifics, just kill any and every invader indiscriminately. Contrast this with the Th2 system, which is the humoral immune system. The Th2 system is responsible for the production of antibodies in the immune system. Think of the Th2 system as the artillery. This is your immune system setting a laser guide on a specific target for the artillery to hit. This system is very specific, very direct and very precise. Therefore the Th2 creates less collateral damage than the Th1.

Just as generals in the field need the ability to coordinate their defenses, these diverse systems also need a form of communication. It is this form of communication, whether short lived or long-term that results in inflammation. This language is via what are called cytokines. Cytokines are in and of themselves not bad. Cytokines are how the body directs the immune system. For example, in the presence of a paper cut, the Th1 system will predominate resulting in an increase in IL-12, IL-2, and IFN-gamma to actively recruit and fight potential infection. It is just when the control of the cytokines is lost or the cytokines are directed against self, that they cause harm. Cytokines are directly involved in inflammation. The cytokines of the Th1 and Th2 systems are different. The Th1 cytokines consist of IL-12, IL-1b, IL-1, and IFN-gamma. The Th2 cytokines consist of IL-4, IL-5, IL-6, IL-10, and IL-13. When balanced, a well functioning immune system is the result. When imbalanced, the result is disease, such as any autoimmune disease.

How does inflammation effect Testosterone? Primarily through estrogen production. Two mechanisms are involved here. Remember that estrogen inhibits testosterone production at the level of the hypothalamus and pituitary. The predominate source of estrogen in men today is aromatase activity in adipose tissue. First, inflammation contributes to low T by increasing aromatase activity (enzyme that converts Testosterone to Estradiol) in adipose tissue (fat) which, in turn, results in more estrogen production. Second, Inflammation contributes to an increase in total adipose tissue. How? Inflammation causes insulin signaling disruption at the GLUT4 receptor. This disruption in insulin signaling results in insulin resistance. Insulin resistance is a "pre-diabetic" condition and is associated with increased adipose tissue.

Inflammation that is controlled is good. Inflammation that is uncontrolled leads to disease. We have already discussed two above. One may consider low T a disease, what with the increase in all-cause mortality (though I consider it physiologic dysfunction). Second, as discussed above, insulin resistance is in part caused by inflammation. What about other disease states? Inflammation arising from the gut has been shown to be the cause of type II Diabetes. Think about that for a moment. Gut inflammation contributes to metabolic dysfunction that results in a systemic disease called Diabetes.

If that doesn't show you that the body is a dynamic creation and not a linear production line, I don't know what will.

But, what about low Testosterone? Can low Testosterone be associated with disease through inflammation? The answer again is yes. Low Testosterone in men has shown to be associated with an increase risk of Lupus and scleroderma in men. The exact mechanism is unknown, but we do know that low Testosterone is associated with increased inflammatory cytokine signaling. We are also aware that low T is associated with a change in the estrogen receptors (ER) from the beta form to alpha form. The ER alpha form promotes an inflammatory signal from the estrogen signal. And what is a prominent cause of low Testosterone to begin with in men? Estrogens. So what we have in men is an estrogen dominant environment contributing to low testosterone. The low Testosterone levels increase inflammatory cytokine signaling itself. But, due to the low Testosterone levels, the estrogen receptor status has changed to a more pro-inflammatory interpretation. And what caused the low testosterone to begin with? Estrogen. Scleroderma and Lupus are autoimmune diseases. Autoimmunity is immune activity directed against self. Immune activity guided through cytokines against self.

Low T is associated with inflammation, inflammatory diseases and increased autoimmune disease. Then the replacement of physiologic levels of Testosterone, should reduce inflammation. That is in fact the case [71]. The chapter on inflammation will dive deeper into the interaction between testosterone and inflammatory signaling.

## Toxins

You hear this word a lot these days. Many proclaim them as the source of most of our health problems today. Others say their

---

71  Kelly DM, Jones TH. Testosterone: a vascular hormone in health and disease. J Endocrinol. June 1 2013;217:R47-R71.

impact is mere overreaction by paranoid individuals. I fall some-where between. I believe that toxins are clearly an obstacle to health, but the impact is predicated by the individuals biochemical system. If they are in a good state of health our own bodies can remove the toxins they are exposed too, then to will manage fine. However, there are some who genetically cannot appropriately manage extra toxin exposure. Plus, environmental toxins are everywhere and the prevalence is increasing.

So what is a toxin? Reminds me of the "Noah" skit by the comedian Bill Cosby, where God is talking to him about building an ark. In one exchange, Noah (Bill Cosby) says what's a cubit? And God responds, "let me see, a cubit, I used to know what a cubit was..." If you haven't heard that skit, you need too; it's great and it's a classic! But I digress. Most, when asked to name toxins, will respond with air and water pollutants, water and food additives... More specifically, environmental toxins are heavy metals, DDT, Bisphenol A, pthalates, parabenes and the like. The toxins that most of us are aware of and the toxins we discuss are of this environmental variety, whether in the general context of pollutants and additives or specific compounds such as DDT and Bisphenol A.

But Webster defines a toxin differently. A toxin is defined by Webster's dictionary as a poisonous substance that is a specific product of the metabolic activity of a living organism. So, a toxin can actually be a product of normal biochemical function. And if a toxin is a product of normal functioning, then our bodies must have biochemical ways to manage them. And of course, the answer is yes.

Detoxification is defined as the ability to remove a harmful substance and/or toxin. A better biochemical definition of detoxification is a chemical change of a xenobiotic, phytochemical and/or endogenous compound into a non-toxic, excretable compound. This definition covers both bases. Whether the toxins are of endogenous source or environmental, the detoxification process is designed to protect and excrete them from the body. The problem is when the body is unable to excrete them. That is the reason that some people don't handle toxin exposures as well as others.

The body uses an incredibly complex detoxification system. One example is the liver. The liver uses a Phase I and Phase II system to handle any endogenous/exogenous toxins. Phase I is a cytochrome P450 dominant process. These are the enzymes that handle this first step. The cytochrome P450 enzymes, 3A4, 1B1, and 1A1 are a few examples. A little note, 50% of prescription drugs use the cytochrome P450 3a4 (CYP3A4) pathway. No wonder people that take 5 or 10 prescriptions don't feel well. It is simply a bottle-neck effect. A lot of drugs trying to going through the same door will create a bottle-neck and slow the detoxification pathways. Just think of traffic. In a traffic jam, you will still get to the destination. However, it will take a lot longer and with an increase risk of disruption and accidents along the way.

Phase II is an amino acid dependent process, with acetylation, sulphation, methylation, and glucuronidation dominating the nomenclature. But that is not the end of it. There can be toxic intermediates that are the product of phase I. And if phase II is not up to the challenge, then oxidative stress is the result. This is where the likes of Glutathione comes in. Glutathione is probably the most potent detoxifier the body makes. Glutathione depletion is a prerequisite for Parkinson's and Alzheimer's disease. And if you unfortunately take too much tylenol, your friendly neighbor ER physician will give you NAC to save your liver from failure. N-acetyl-glutathione, as it is known, is the precursor to glutathione.

Now, according to the FDA, detoxification doesn't exist. A recent statement from the FDA in August of 2012 **commanded** google disable adword accounts of nutritional supplement companies that advertised chelation and detoxification. Here, the FDA treated detoxification as merely an advertising or grammar problem. What's next, do physicians need to be worried about hanging participles? (What is a hanging participle, I use to know what a hanging participle was....) However, what the FDA fails to recognize is that every cell of the body must detoxify. Detoxification is critical to health and a prerequisite for disease. The primary organs of detoxification are the liver, kidneys, skin, lungs, and the gut. Can anyone live without the ability to detoxify? Can anyone live without their liver?

All this highlights the importance of limiting toxin exposure from our environment. If we are already producing toxins as a part of our day to day functioning, how is the extra toxic burden going to impact our bodies biochemical ability to handle more?. And thus we see another factor in the health decline today.

For the purpose of the discussion that follows, when we refer to toxins, we are referring to the environmental variety.

First, is there even a problem with environmental toxins? Yes. Not only are we being exposed to toxins with every passing day, but we are exposed while still in our mother's womb. This is how we are seeing such drastic changes in health. Our genes are not changing, but the expression of our genes are. That is how from one generation to the next, a drastic change can manifest. Changes to the genetic code take thousands of years, but change in expression, take just a generation.

But how do toxins effect testosterone? Most environmental toxins have estrogenic activity. Most environmental toxins are better known as xenoestrogens. A xenoestrogen is of course not an estrogen. But the xenoestrogen binds to the same receptor as the estrogens and the signal is interpreted as if it were an estrogen itself.

Whether they are pesticides, insecticides or you name it, they signal as if an estrogen.

How about a few examples? Let's look at Bisphenol A and two effects described in the scientific literature. A 2007 study found that Bisphenol A changed the Estrogen receptor expression from beta form to alpha form, in the offspring born to the female rats exposed [72]. So, maternal exposure, altered the physiology of the unborn rat. But, of course that is rats. How about humans? A 2006 study, found Bisphenol A to be present in small levels in pregnant mothers and even in their unborn child. As small as these levels were, they still exceeded the levels at which receptors change occurs as the result of BPA exposure[73]. So, this study showed that Bisphenol A exposure is detected at levels at which change occurs even before birth. The newborn child's physiology is changed though unborn.

## Medications

That is right. What is said about the problem? That the cause of the problem is usually staring you right in the face. No where is this more evident than in the case of prescription drugs. The third leading cause of death today is? Drum role please....prescription drugs, drug to drug interactions, and medical procedures. Let me repeat that. The 3rd leading cause of death today is due to prescription drugs and their interactions. I thought there was something called the Hypocratic oath?

We physicians and other medical providers have been lulled into believing that because it is prescribed by us (physicians and other

---

72  Monje L et al. Neonatal exposure to bisphenol A modifies the abundance of estrogen receptor alpha transcripts with alternative 5-untranslated regions in the female rat preoptic area. J Endocrinol. July 1 2007;194:201-212.

73  Welshons WV, Nagel SC, Saal FS. Large effects from small exposure. III. Endocrine Mechanisms mediating effects of Bisphenol A at levels of human exposure. Endocrinology. Jun 1 2006;147(6):s56-s69.

medical providers), it is safe and without out risk. A recent report found that 70% of Americans are taking one daily medication and 25% are taking 4 daily prescription medications [74].

But of course, there are risks, even major complications and/or death? Patients too have been lulled into the belief that prescription drugs are inherently safe, without complications. Everybody would rightly question the prescription use of heroin or cocaine due to it's risk and inherent addiction capacity. (Believe it or not, both were at one time FDA approved drugs.) But few question the massive increase in pre-scriptive use of benzodiazepines and anti-depressants. The use of anti-depressant use has increased 400% over the last 20 years. These carry very similar addiction risks and equally dangerous side effects. The black box label on anti-depressants declare an increase risk of suicide. No greater risk than that. By the way, New York state is now confiscating guns from those who are taking anti-depressants.

But, this is about testosterone. Obviously, physicians are not going to prescribe Estradiol for a man. Let's look at very commonly pre-scribed medication today. Few drugs are more prescribed than the class of drugs called statins. Statin drugs are prescribed to lower cho-lesterol. Here is the perfect example of the problem starring right at you. A 2010 study showed that statin drugs lower testosterone levels in men[75]. Here is the dichotomy of this situation. The statin therapy is prescribed to reduce cholesterol and reduce cardiovascular disease risk: prevent stroke, heart attacks...But, the same statin therapy has been shown to reduce testosterone levels in men. And may I remind you, that low Testosterone levels are associated with an increase risk in all-cause mortality in men, especially cardiovascular.

---

74  Kottke TE. Reversing the slide in US health outcomes and deteriorating health care economics. Mayo Clinic Proceedings. June 2013;88(6):533-535.

75  Giovanni Corona et al. The effect of statin therapy on Testosterone levels in Subjects consulting for Erectile Dysfunction. The Journal of Sexual Medicine. April 2010;(7):1547-1556.

## Hormone therapy

That is right. I propose that testosterone therapy should be the last thing done for men with low Testosterone. A lot of you may be asking why? If you review everything that we have been discussing about the causes of low Testosterone, you will see why. Low Testosterone is usually the end effect and not the cause. So, with any problem, if you correct the cause at it's source, then the effect will be solutions with minimal side effects.

For too long, medicine has been chasing its tail after symptoms. Traditional medicine (and I am a traditionally trained MD) does a great job of detecting and/or managing diseases. But if your goal is health and wellness, then you need to change your perspective. What medicine should be doing is using the symptoms and/or physical signs to help direct them where to look. I say look for the cause. The cause is the source of the problem. Now, one caveat. Not all problems have causes that can be fixed. Sometimes things are broken or dysfunction has gone on for far too long and the point of no return has passed. But that is rare. The body is designed to heal itself. Some paths are just easier than others. But that requires time and a different paradigm of medicine. A different focus. A different model of the patient:physician ratio. A different topic for a different book.

A man with high estrogens (Estrone/Estradiol) as the cause of low Testosterone, which I propose is a majority, is just throwing fuel on the fire by starting on Testosterone. The cause in this case would be the high aromatase activity and the resultant estrogen dominance. The effect is low Testosterone. I have seen this far too often. Forty something man presents to physician for "low T" symptoms. He is started on testosterone therapy. He does great for a few months, but then starts to notice some urinary voiding problems. Presents to his Urologist and is found to have a significant increase in his PSA value. The testosterone is converted to estrogen which bumps the PSA level. The next step is biopsy and/or prescription and/or surgery.

This was exactly the case of a client that came to see us. He was on testosterone therapy prescribed by me, but he was feeling so good he thought he would just increase his dosing to his personal liking. His initial PSA on first visit was 2.1. He presented to a local ER after 10 weeks post self dosing, with significant urinary voiding problems. He was diagnosed with prostatitis and instructed to visit his Urologist. The urologist added more antibiotics to the ones he was already taking from the ER and checked his PSA. The PSA had jumped to 10. That is a big jump for a PSA. Antibiotics did nothing to fix the problem. We re-evaluated his androgens and estrogens. His self-dosing had caused his estrogen levels to spike. Intensive therapy to lower his estrogen production resolved his prostate problem and his PSA on last check was 1.2. All the result of inappropriate testosterone therapy.

We need a change in medicine. We need a change in paradigm. It has been said, "where your treasure is, therefore is your heart". We need a change in heart in medicine. We need to refocus on the causes of the problem rather than simply treating the symptoms. No place is this more evident, than in men with Low T.

# CHAPTER 5

# SOLUTIONS

It is always amazing what we find ourselves doing at the end of each year. The years just seem to fly by. We wake up to January 1 of each new year resolving to do something new, to do something better, to change something…we all take the plunge into the New Year's resolution. Some, more successful than others.

But, why the need for resolutions? Because we need solutions.

The need for a resolution implies that a problem exists. That we need a change of direction. With the resolution, we have a resolve or determination to do something better. We are focusing on solutions rather than the problems. We feel the need for solutions to fix the prior year of band aids and the lack of resolution they gave.

No where is this solutions-based focus more needed than in the battle for our health.

To find solutions, we must define the problem. The problem is our current disease model doesn't work for health or health restoration.

It does do a good job of managing disease. But, not resolving it. If your focus is on containing or managing disease, then that is exactly what you will do. Health or wellness doesn't just happen. You have to focus on it.

So, what does the research say in reply to the above statement?

The future of the health of Americans is bleak. According to a recent article from the Lancet[76], 50% of Americans will be obese by the year 2030 (obesity defined as BMI 30). The same article showed that 13 states have an obesity rate exceeding 30% now, when in the year 2000, no states had an obesity rate exceeding 30%. The healthiest state was Colorado, but it's obesity rate just clipped the 20% mark. In fact, no state had an obesity rate 20%. Another article from the journal Obesity[77], revealed that 86% of American adults will be obese or overweight by 2030. Of course, these are projections based on recent historical trends. But the point is that the trajectory is headed in the wrong direction.

But, we don't have to wait until 2030. According to the Organization for Economic Cooperation and Development (OECD), 75% of Americans will be obese or overweight (overweight defined as BMI 25 and 30) by 2020. And it is worse for men, where 82% are estimated to be obese or overweight.

What is the Impact? According to the International Diabetes Federation Foundation in 2011, 1 in 10 adults will have diabetes by 2030. That equates to 552 million adults worldwide. That is a startling number of people with Diabetes. Again, according to the OECD, money spent/lost on of obesity in the US has reached an estimated 1% of GDP.

---

76  Urgently needed: a framework convention for obesity control. The Lancet. August 27 2011;9793(378):741.

77  Wang Y et al. Will all Americans become overweight or obese? Estimating the progression and cost of the US obesity epidemic. Oct 2008;16(10):2323-2330.

Where has our current disease-medical paradigm gotten us in the obesity battle? If you look at the statistics, nowhere. In fact, we are losing the battle. Yet, we continue to pour money down a failing medical model, for obesity, that studies have shown just doesn't work.

What we need is a solutions based approach to the obesity epidemic. We need a resolution to do better as a medical community. We need a resolution to focus on solutions, not band-aids. We need a resolution to focus on health and health restoration: not on disease management.

Why the focus on obesity? Obesity is one of the biggest contributors to low T in men. Low T in men equals poor health.

I'm biased, I feel that this solutions based medicine is provided through the integrative medical movement today. But, I see integrative medicine falling prey to the same follies that plagues traditional medicine. Don't get them all the way well, but closer than traditional medicine; and be more natural about it, because it is safer. Keep them coming back for follow ups, because we need those appointments. Use the same one-size-fits-all approach that traditional medicine does, just do it more naturally. This is a constant battle for integrative practitioners, for all practitioners, and yes I struggle with this too.

Why? Because it is what we are taught.

But some people don't desire solutions (seen our government lately?). They don't desire wellness. Health is a choice. These individuals take comfort in their illness, their disease, their brokeness.

Reminds me of a female client that I saw that was "stressed out". I know this book is about men and their testosterone, but this example supports my point. Her history revealed a long history of extreme stress with a spike preceding her appointment. We discussed options for evaluation and the purpose for evaluation. She agreed to this plan and we would await her results to start treatment based on her biochemical test results. However, I received an e-mail 24 hours later. The client was very upset that I had not written her an anti-depressant, despite her agreeing to the management plan. This was one of my "head banging" moments. This client did not want a path to wellness, she just wanted a quick-fix in a pill. This client was used to the band-aid approach.

Many describe a state of "welfare". A generational way of life that becomes embedded in one's psyche that is extremely difficult to break. Just like a heroin addict, the dependency is comfortable and the change is difficult. I look a lot at what health care promotes today as what I call "diseasefare". What?!?! Stay with me... Traditional medicine perpetuates a generational state of disease. There is no incentive for healing. If one actually gets well, there will be no return clients. No follow up in 2 weeks. No full schedule. There must be no wellness so that there can be follow up appointments.

The first time these thoughts came to me, I thought, "no way". It felt like a conspiracy theory. Now, after practicing integrative medicine for 8 years, I say: "yeah, that's about right".

The diseasefare defines the person. It provides them a way of living. It promotes dependancy. A dependency on the system. Why would you want to break it. It is in someways easy, because it requires no change.

You see this in families. There seems to be a perpetual disease or illness mentality. For example, the mother who was diagnosed with fibromyalgia at a young age requiring multiple medications. Then her daughter or son get diagnosed at a similar young age with the same fibromyalgia and the same treatment. It is as if they have their class. Not a upper, middle, or lower class; but a disease class. It has become their lot in life. Because not a lot of effort is required.

I know what I said sounds harsh, but it is true. Some people do not want to be well. I have seen it first hand. I spent many years banging my head against the wall trying to help people be well that had no desire to leave their state of disease. It was like their best friend. And they couldn't turn their back on their best friend now could they? Worse yet, it was who they were. Too break free from disease would require a fresh start...a clean slate. Now that is difficult. A fresh start, a clean state, the unknown. At least the disease is known. It is who they are.

As Hippocrates said, "Healing in a matter of time, but it is sometimes also a matter of opportunity". Sadly, some people bypass the opportunity to achieve health, because they just don't have time or the effort required to change course. Only in the presence of disease, is the value of health realized.

Enough bashing the problem. On to solutions!

Solutions requires some structure. At Seasons we work to achieve customized health and wellness by following the 5 points of Wellness. Below is a brief explanation of the 5 points of Wellness that we follow at Seasons. We will then broaden and deepen our discussion of each in the subsequent chapters.

## NUTRITION

We are what we eat. More than that, we are what our body does with what we eat. Hippocrates said it best, "Let food be your medicine and medicine be your food". But that food must be customized. Nutrition must be individualized to meet your metabolic needs, limit inflammatory responses, and meet your lifestyle demands.

Sure it would be easy to be able to say Paleo for all, Atkins for everyone or wheat belly for life? Sure they are good recommendations and will help men, but that will not work for everyone. Is it any wonder why 98% of weight loss programs fail? It is because they are one-size-fits-all approach. Whatever name you give to the program, a one-size-fits-all approach doesn't cut it. This holds true whether your using a traditional medical model or an integrative medical model.

Individual nutritional counseling is a staple with our clients. We want to meet your individual nutritional needs in a way that fits you lifestyle.

## EXERCISE

We can't do without it! Exercise is the means to burn calories. Yes, more calories out than in helps maintain healthy weight. But exercise does so much more. Exercise builds muscle. Exercise relieves stress. Exercise helps to detoxify. However, too much exercise can severely harm the body. So, Exercise must meet metabolic demands as much as your ability and time allows.

At Seasons, we work to maximize your calorie expenditure, while reducing the damage to your body from excessive exercise. We do this in a way to match your lifestyle and your physical abilities.

In many individuals, I will actually restrict their exercise in the initial phases of treatment. Why? Testing had revealed their body's metabolism is in no place to handle the rigors of even a small work out.

As with diet, it would be easy and great if all could train for a marathon or do p90X. However, most don't want to; nor do they even need to.

## HORMONES

Sexy topic these days. Doesn't matter your age, you need hormones. Hormones are a means of communication of your body. They are the message. It is not just about individual hormones, it is about balance. Sure it would be great if men were just a Testosterone sponge; or women just an Estrogen factory. That is what the marketing mantra says (instead of evidence-based physicians, we physicians have allowed ourselves to become marketing-mantra based physicians). But, of course, the balance of all the hormones is the key to health. Just look at your body, we are a creation of balance. When your hormones are balanced, so are you. When your hormones are not balanced, your body will let you know–called symptoms.

Your hormone balance is unique to you. And you can bet it will change. The only way to determine your imbalance is to listen to your symptoms to direct your provider where to look. Only then can you identify your particular imbalance and formulate a plan to balance your hormones. This will include bioidentical hormone therapy (BHRT). Like for like. Why would a physician give you provera (medroxypregesterone acetate), when your body wants progesterone? Would you give your child sour grapes? Of course not. It's still grapes, they have just gone sour. Give the body what it wants; in the form it wants, in the safest delivery method to balance the hormones. This, and only this way, can hormones be balanced. Balanced hormones equals health and wellness.

Again, I see too many medical providers roll the traditional medical model into a quasi integrative model. It is just more "natural". What is natural about giving the body what it needs. That is just right!

## INFLAMMATION

Inflammation is the great obstacle to health and wellness. Inflammation is a part of the bodies immune system signaling. Pain, redness, swelling, heat, and loss of function are common manifestations of inflammation. Inflammation is not new. Inflammation is as old as Adam and Eve. The first description of the four classical signs of inflammation were described by Celsius (30 BC – 38 AD).

The source of inflammation is going to be unique to each person. It may be due to deficiencies, such as vitamin D deficiencies or could be due to poor dietary intake of antioxidants, such as resveratrol and curcumin. It could even be due to dietary deficiency of fish. Low Omega-3 intake leads to inflammation. Just look at Americans today. Part of our problem today, in the US, is the Sad American Diet. In most cases, our inflammation is the result of our diet.

Or the inflammation could be coming from your gut! Did you know that up to 75% of your immune system lines your gut? In many ways, your health starts with your gut. Look to where your body puts most of its defenses to find the major source of inflammation.

As you can see, the source of inflammation is as different as the individual. The only way to identify the individual's unique source of inflammation is to listen to the body. The body will tell you or show you what and where the source is. Then it is up to your provider to find the causes and implement specific therapy to eliminate inflammation. This can be as diverse as parasite treatment to simple dietary changes.

## DETOXIFICATION

To steal from Nike's slogan, "just do it". We have to just do it. Detoxify that is.

Many will call it cleansing. Others may refer to it as metabolization. But, whatever one calls it, it cannot be found in a bottle. It occurs in the body. It is complex, individualized and needs evaluation to determine needed support.

We live in a toxic world today. There is no way around that! According to a recent study, detectable levels of toxins were found in up to 99% of pregnant women[78]. Many of these chemicals have been banned since the early 1970's. And this number will only rise with the approximately 1,800 new chemicals approved annually. And according to the ATSDR, more than 80,000 chemicals are currently in our environment today, with the previously mentioned 1,800 added annually. You don't have to be a liberal, in the political spectrum, to see that our environment is impacting our health. Health is not a political issue.

According to the World Health Organization, 24% of disease can be contributed to toxin exposure. This tidal wave of toxins are overwhelming our detoxifications systems. To protect ourselves against this toxin onslaught, every cell in our bodies must detoxify. Just look to the exponential rise in the rates of autism spectrum disorder and neurodegenerative diseases, such as Alzheimer's, Parkinson's, and MS. And no, this has nothing to do with better testing. These disease are on the rise. Yet, few bother to wonder why.

The ability to detoxify is critical to health. Our focus at Seasons is to evaluate your individual ability to detoxification and remedy those areas that are dysfunctional. We focus on your major detox organs: liver, skin, kidneys, lymphatics, and GI tract, though every cell in the body must detoxify. Then we provide a detoxification plan to meet your specific toxic load and to support your identified detoxification needs.

As you can see, symptom based therapy need not apply. Use your symptoms to identify the source of the problem(s). Individual therapy directed at the source is the only way to provide Health and Wellness.

---

78   Woodruff TJ, Zota AR, Schwartz JM. Environmental Chemicals in Pregnant Women in the United States: NHANES 2003-2004. Environ Health Perspect. June 2011;119(6):878-885.

It was Aristotle who said, " the whole is more than the sum of its parts". Or as Hippocrates said, "treat the body as a whole, rather than the sum of its parts".

Health is a choice. Health is an opportunity. Don't miss your opportunity to choose a Health and Wellness Lifestyle. Unfortunately, many do. Not because they missed the turn, but because they chose to.

# CHAPTER 6

# NUTRITION

Truth without Corruption. Corruption of the truth permeates health care today. What does this have to do with men's health? Everything. The corruption in health today, is the perpetuated truth that health can be achieved through a pill. The corruption in health today, is that obesity is the result of God forgetting to bypass your stomach. The corruption in health today, is that weight loss does not require lifestyle change. That health can be achieved without nutrition. The truth is, health, or lack of health begins with nutrition. Any statement to the contrary is void of truth or a complete lack of knowledge.

Effective weight loss can only be achieved through targeted Wellness through nutrition.

I recently met a man that works for a pharmaceutical company. I asked him what he does in his role as he was not a pharmaceutical rep. He told me that he works with a health insurance company in the south, particularly Louisiana. I won't give out the name, but the first letter is B and the last S. Of course, that caught my attention, so I asked him what exactly he did. Get this. This gentleman was employed by the pharmaceutical company and he consulted with the medical directors of this health insurance company to write position statements. What are position statements? Position statements are the published policies that determine the health insurance coverage of medical services. These are statements supposedly created in the bowels of scientific scrutiny, but in this case, in the presence of conflicts of interest. This case shows the corruption of the health care system today. Your physicians coverage of a treatment/diagnostic test by this health insurance company could very well have been defined by this health insurance company consulting with a pharmaceutical company which provides the means of therapy.

No scientific scrutiny. No truth. Just corruption. You scratch my back, I stuff your back wallet.

Obesity is the number #1 health problem today. By health problem, I mean obstacle to health. As I have said many times, obesity is the doorway to disease. Sixty-seven percent of Americans are either overweight or obese today. And for the first time, people that are obese exceed those that are overweight. According to a CDC 2009 report, approximately, 34% of Americans were estimated to be obese in 2005/2006. That equated to 72 million people. Actual 2011 statistics by the CDC reveal an obesity rate of 35.7% [79]. The numbers are not improving either. The same data from the CDC found that thirteen states have an obesity rate over 30%. Two points that are very concerning about that. First, there were ZERO states with obesity rates exceeding 30% in the year 2000. Second, these states are not just barely exceeding 30%. For example, the obesity rate of Mississippi was at 34.9%. The slope of change over the past 11 years is accelerating. This acceleration is going in the wrong direction. These states are already on the fast track to 40%.

---

79   from http://www.cdc.gov/obesity/data/adult.html.

The state that I used to practice in, Louisiana, and the state that I currently practice in, Tennessee, are unfortunately at the top of this list as well.

What about our future? Look to our children.

More children battle obesity today than ever before. The statistics in children are alarming, with up to 17% of children and adolescents being obese [80]. Worse yet, this is a 3 fold increase in one generation. Metabolic syndrome is the result of obesity. I discussed the criteria of metabolic syndrome in chapter 1.

In review, Metabolic syndrome consists of 3 of the 5 following criteria:

- Blood pressure ≥ 130/85
- Abdominal circumference > 40 inches
- Triglycerides ≥ 150
- HDL < 40
- Fasting glucose ≥ 110

Metabolic syndrome was once considered an adult disease only, yet now metabolic syndrome is booming in children [81]. The prevalence of metabolic syndrome is 39.7% in moderately obese children and 49.7% in severely obese children [82]. As obesity goes, so goes metabolic syndrome. As metabolic syndrome goes, so goes disease.

---

80  http://www.cdc.gov/about/grand-rounds/archives/2010/06-June.htm

81  Alberti KG et al. Harmonizing the metabolic syndrome: a joint interim statement of the International Diabetes Federation Task Force on Epidemiology and Prevention: National Heart, Lung, and Blood Institute; American Heart Association;World Heart Federation; International Atherosclerosis Society; and International Association for the Study of Obesity. Circulation. 2009;120:1640-1645.

82  Weiss R et al. Obesity and the Metabolic Syndrome in Children and Adolescents. N Engl J Med. 2004;350:2362-2374.

We as a nation need to improve our health. To improve health we must focus on health, embracing a wellness model instead of a disease model. This starts by losing weight. But we need to lose weight the right way. Actually, helping people lose weight is not that difficult, but helping people lose weight and maintain the weight loss proves to be much more difficult. If it was easy, everybody would do it.

So, how to fix the problem? Medicine and others are not short of ways to attempt weight loss. However, it has been estimated that 95% of weight loss programs fail. These programs do not fail at weight loss, they fail at sustaining weight loss. They are short on solutions in sustained weight loss. Remember, the obesity epidemic is the foundation of our health crisis today.

Just look around. There are weight loss "gimmicks" all over the place. According to the free dictionary, a gimmick is defined as "a device employed to cheat, deceive, or trick..." Gimmicks come in all forms: from prepackaged meals, to protein shakes, to prescription drugs (see adipex, xenical, belviq...), to the newest gimmicks–HCG and weight loss surgeries. All these gimmicks have one thing in common–failure. Yes, they will help you lose some weight, but they fail miserably in the maintenance department. Thus, you keep shopping your weight loss programs to the detriment of your metabolism. This technique actually makes your long-term weight loss that much more difficult and destroy your health.

Don't think that the "medical" weight loss programs are any better. If your program isn't based on your individual metabolism, as determined by testing, then your program is a gimmick.

Let's look at a few examples. First, adipex is a commonly prescribed drug that helps people lose weight. It is an amphetamine-like compound that speeds up the metabolism and suppresses the appetite. It works great short-term. However, without lifestyle change rebound will occur. The rebound is worse with adipex because it alters the body's ability to lose weight. Adipex does this through muscle loss and thyroid dysfunction. Oh, and did I forget to mention addiction. There are even addiction clinics for those on adipex?! To see the addiction capacity of adipex, look to the very common amphetamine–methamphetamine or by its street name–Meth. How many mug shots of people on Meth have you seen that are obese? None. They all lose weight. But, they lose weight at the expense of a horrible addiction.

And the new comers on the block is HCG (Human Chorionic Gonadotropin) and weight loss surgery. Really, whose cause of obesity is an HCG deficiency? HCG is at its highest level of production in women during pregnancy. I know you don't think of pregnancy as a way to lose weight (And of course, it is not). In fact, a woman's metabolism promotes weight gain during pregnancy. Then, throw in the fact that the "HCG diet" calls for only 500 calories daily. That is nothing other than starvation. This starvation will actually slow your thyroid function and trigger a slowing of metabolism in the long term. Thus when you come off the HCG and the 500 cal diet, rebound weight gain occurs. And who can maintain a 500 cal diet?

What does the science say about the HCG diet? What does the science say? Not what does opinion say. The scientific literature tells us everything we need to know about HCG. The HCG component of the diet doesn't work. Sure, 500 calories a day helps one lose weight. That is classified as starvation. The question is: does the HCG component plus the 500 calorie/day diet provide weight loss beyond that of a 500 calorie diet alone?

The study that started it all was published in 1954 by Simeons AT [83]. This was the first study to show benefit of HCG in those on

---

[83]  Simeons AT. The action of chorionic gonadotrophin in the obese. Lancet. Nov 6 1954;267(6845):946-7.

500 calorie/day diets above those on 500 calorie/day diet alone. This was referred to as the Simeons theory. Several studies were subsequently done and some found benefit and others found no benefit. However, these studies were small and inconclusive. In 1973, Asher and Harper duplicated the original study and found benefit of HCG above 500 calorie/day diet alone in 20 patients [84]. However, subsequent duplication of the Asher and Harper studies found no benefit from the addition of HCG [85 86 87 88 89]. Several studies have actually shown weight gain with HCG [90] [91]. A meta-analysis of 24 studies in 1995 came to the conclusion that "there is no scientific evidence that HCG is effective in the treatment of obesity; it does not bring about weight-loss of fat-redistribution, nor does it reduce hunger or induce a feeling of well-being" [92]. Include the suggestion in the scientific literature

84 Asher WL, Harper HW. Effect of human chorionic gonadotrophin on weight loss, hunger, and feeling of well-being. Am J Clin Nutr. 1973;26:211.

85 Young RL, Fuchs RJ, Woltien MJ. Chorionic gonadotropin in weight control A double-blind crossover study. JAMA. Nov 29 1976;236(22): 2495-7.

86 Stein MR et al Ineffectiveness of huan chorionic gonadotropin in weight reduction: a double-blind study. Am J Clin Nutr. Sept 1976;29(9):940-8.

87 Greenway FL, Bray GA. Human chorionic gonadotropin (HCG) in the treatment of obesity: a critical assessment of the Simeons method. West J Med. Dec 1977;127(6):461-3.

88 Miller R, Schneiderman LJ. A clinical study of the use of human chorionic gonadotrophin in weight reduction. J Fam Pract. Mar 1977;4(3):445-8.

89 Bosch B et al. Human chorionic gonadotropin and weight loss. A double-blind, placebo-controlled trial. S Afr Med J. Feb 17 1990;77(4):185-9.

90 Parkash SG et al. Phase I study of human chorionic gonadotropin given subcutaneously to patients with acquired immunodeficiency syndrome-related mucocutaneous Kaposi's Sarcoma. J Natl Cancer Inst. 1997;89(23):1797-1802.

91 Rippel RH, Johnson ES. Inhibition of HCG-induced ovarian and uterine weight augmentation in the immature rat by analogs. Proc Soc Exp Biol Med. Jul 1976;152(3):432-6.

92 Lijesen GK et al. The effect of human chorionic gonadotropin (HCG) in the treatment of obesity by means of the Simeons therapy: a criteria-based meta-analysis. Br J Clin Pharmacol. Sept 1995;40(3):237-243.

of a link between HCG and autoimmune disease [93] [94] [95], and there is no valid reproducible scientific evidence or metabolic reason for HCG for weight loss.

And the worst gimmick of all are the weight-loss surgeries. Let's objectively think about this. Who can realistically say that their weight problem is the result of a stomach that is too large? I think our creator knew what he was doing when he made our gastrointestinal system. I don't believe that God forgot a bypass or sleeve around the stomach. Let's run with that logic for a moment. Are headaches the result of a lack of a lobotomy. Is diabetic neuropathy is due to the lack of amputee of the effected limb. Sounds ridiculous doesn't it. But that is where our logic is today with regards to weight loss treatment. We accept the ridiculous and ridicule the logical.

We need to look at weight loss differently. Our goals should not be weight loss itself. Excess weight is a symptom just like fatigue or insomnia. If, I help people lose weight in an unhealthy way, one that does not maintain weight loss, have I done anything good by that approach? No. All I have done is hurt the individual and contribute to the 98.8% failure rate. Instead, the focus should be on Health and Wellness. Weight loss will come as a by-product of healthier living. That is weight loss the right way. And of course it begins with nutrition. Nutrition is the corner stone of a healthy lifestyle. Nutrition is a corner stone of the treatment of low Testosterone.

Why is weight loss and healthy living so difficult? Because each individual has unique genetics and a unique metabolic signature.

---

93  Thau RB et al. Failure of gonadotropin therapy secondary to chorionic gonadotropin-induced antibodies. J Clin Endocrinol Metab. Apr 1988;66(4):862-7.

94  Sokol RZ et al. Gonadotropin therapy failure secondary to human chorionic gonadotropin-induced antibodies. J Clin Endocr Metab. May 1981;52(5):929-32.

95  Ogura T et al. Hypothyroidism associated with anti-human chorionic gonadotropin antibodies secondarily produced by gonadotropin therapy in a case of idiopathic hypothalamic hypogonadism. J Endocrinol Invest. Nov 2003;26(11):1128-35.

Each individual's road to obesity is different. Thus their roadmap to weight-loss and health will be equally unique. Some will have hypothyroidism. Some will have insulin resistance. Yes, some don't exercise. All will have inflammation. But these alone will not explain the accelerating obesity rates documented above. Sorry, it is not as simple as calories in and calories out.

I love to use analogies to make things stick. My dad is a commercial pilot for a major airline. When we were discussing this book, he said, "Nathan, there is no perfect flight". His point was, there is always going to be something that goes wrong. Whether it is a ground delay, a flight deviation, or computer glitch—something will always go wrong. Rarely, does something catastrophically go wrong. He has only had to declare an emergency three times in his 40 years of flying. But, the pilot is to be there to handle things when they do go wrong. To do that, the pilot must have an excellent working knowledge of the systems of the his/her airplane and the procedures required to solve the problem, should one arise.

Take that analogy and extrapolate it to a physician. Sure, most weight loss programs do not result in major catastrophe (minus weight loss surgeries of course). But, how many weight loss programs fail? According to data and perception , 98.8% of weight loss programs fail. Why do they fail? Is it maybe that the "pilot" (physician) doesn't know the internal workings of the "plane" (body) and does not know what the body needs to right the metabolic ship? Restated, the medical provider doesn't understand the internal biochemical dysfunction that negatively effects the metabolism and causes weight gain. The average physician functions at a level that is far behind that of the current scientific knowledge. According to an Institute of Medicine Report[96], it takes an aver-

---

96  Institute of Medicine Committee on Quality of Health Care in America. *Crossing the Quality Chasm: A New Health System for the 21st Century*. Washington, DC: National Academy Press, 2001, p 364.

age of 17 years for new scientific knowledge to reach integration in the clinical practice. We shouldn't be surprised that when no weight loss occurs, or when the client plateaus' or even starts to gain weight, the often subtle changes needed go unchanged due to a lack of working knowledge.

Let's get down to the basics.

There can be many causes of poor health and most involve nutrition. There can be genetic influences, macronutrient imbalances (proteins, carbohydrates, fats), and there can be micronutrient deficiencies, and there can be overnutrition–all of which are nutrition based problems. There can also be hormone imbalances, inflammation, detoxification, and mitochondrial disruption. Let's first focus on the nutritional-based causes: genetics, macronutrient and micronutrient components.

Put simply, macronutrients and micronutrients are nutrition. Macronutrients and micronutrients are essential. They are the essence of how the body makes energy. Genetics influence how the body handles the intake of these nutrient building blocks. You are what you eat! You can't have health or disease without it. Nutrition is the foundation for both. But, you get to choose which one.

## Genetics

It has been estimated that 30-40% of obesity has genetics at its origin [97] [98]. This shouldn't surprise us, as we are all created unique. Our genes are the background makeup of who we are individually. Our genetics make up who we are and how we interact with our environment. In turn, the environment is what helps to influence

---

97  Hunt MS et al. Familial resemblance of 7-year changes in body mass and adiposity. Obes Res. 2002;10:507-517.

98  Coady SA et al. Genetic variability of adult body mass index: a longitudinal assessment in Framingham families. Obes Res. 2002;10:675-681.

the manifestation of these genetic tendencies. We are all genetically predisposed to something. No one is immune to that (sorry, no one is going to live forever in this bodily form). This is call epigenetics. Epigenetics is the understanding that genetics and the environment play a role in our health or in our disease state. Nutrition and obesity is no different. Fortunately for us only 30-40% of obesity has a genetic origin. We still have the benefit of the 60-70% that does not have its origin in genetics to effect change and positively influence our health. In most people today, that means weight loss.

But before we leave our the discussion on genetics, let's consider that how our genetics (DNA) influences how we metabolize food. Our genetics encode the ability for our bodies to digest, absorb, and utilize the foods that we eat. Just because our genetics encode a protein that enables us to do these essential functions, does not make the function of that protein perfect. In fact, very small genetic encoding errors can create a ripple effect throughout the metabolism. This is a documented factor in deficient carbohydrate metabolism [99] [100], protein metabolism [101], and fat metabolism [102] [103]. These genetically caused metabolic dysfunctions are the result of Single Nucleotide Polymorphisms (SNPs). These are single encoding errors that cause physiologic dysfunction in the final encoded product. These SNPs or other genetic variants can even influence

99   Eny KM, Wolever TMS, Fontaine-Bisson B, El-Sohemy A. Genetic variant in the glucose transporter type 2 is associated with higher intakes of sugars in two distinct populations. Physiological genomics. Mar 18 2008;33(3):355-360.

100  Dupuis J et al. New genetic loci implicated in fasting glucose homeostasis and their impact on type 2 diabetes risk. Nat Genet. Feb 2010;42(2):105-116.

101  Huuskonen A, Lappalainen J, Oksala N, Santtila M, Hakkinen K, Kyrolainen H, Atalay M. Common genetic variation in the IGF-1 associates with maximal force output. Medicine and Science in Sports and Exercise. 2011;43(12):2368-2374.

102  Warodomwichit D et al. The monosaturated fatty acid intake modulates the effect of ADIPOQ polymorphisms on obesity. Obesity (Silver Spring). Mar 2009;17(3):510-517.

103  Kraja AT et al. Genetic analysis of 16 NMR-Lipoprotein fractions in humans, the GOLDN study. Lipids. Feb 2013;48(2):155-65.

how exercise effects obesity [104], how exercise effects insulin signaling [105], how food is used to reward and influence energy intake [106], and even effect taste [107]. So, one genetic encoding error can influence the level of metabolic benefit provided through exercise or how effectively nutrition is either used or stored. When it comes to nutrition and weight loss today, it is possible for an individual to have customized nutritional counseling and even exercising planning based on their individual genetics.

Balanced Nutrition is always the best nutrition. I often speak of balance when it comes to hormones, but it equally applies to nutrition. The balance I am referring to here is with regards to the macronutrients: proteins, carbohydrates, and fats. Of course, Americans have a very imbalanced diet–high carbohydrate intake relative to proteins and fats. This imbalance has not always been the case. According to the National Health and Nutrition Examination Surveys (NHANES) from 1971 to 2000, carbohydrate intake increased by 62.4 grams in women and 67.7 grams in men, fat intake increased by 6.5 grams in women and decreased by 5.3 grams in men, and protein intake stayed relatively constant [108]. Now compare these stats to the rise in

---

104  Vimaleswaran KS et al. Physical activity attenuates the body mass index-increasing influence of genetic variation in the FTO gene. Am J Clin Nutr. Aug 2009;90(2):425-428.

105  Teran-Garcia M et al. Hepatic lipase gene variant-514CT is associated with lipoprotein and insulin sensitivity response to regular exercise: The HERITAGE family study. Diabetes. Jul 2005;54(7):2251-2255.

106  Epstein LH et al. Food reinforcement, the Dopamin D2 Receptor Genotype, and energy intake in obese and nonobese humans. Behav Neurosci. Oct 2007;121(5):877-886.

107  Kim UK, Jorgenson E, Coon H, Leppert M, Risch N, Drayna D. Positional cloning of the human quantitative trait locus underlying taste sensitivity to phenylthiocarbamide. Science. Feb 21 2003;299(5610):1221-5.

108  Chanmugan P, Guthrie JF, Cecilio S, Morton JF, Basiotis PP, Anand R. Did fat intake in the United States really decline between 1989-1991 and 1994-1996? J Am Diet Assoc. 2003;103:867-72.

obesity from 14.5% to 30.9% over the same time period [109] and a picture of increasing macronutrient imbalance appears.

Of course, this is not the only factor associated with the increase in obesity. But clearly, the rise in carbohydrate intake, particularly refined sugars, has mirrored the rise in the obesity rate. Not all carbohydrates are created equally. The greatest rise in carbohydrate intake is that of refined or simple sugar. The annual sugar intake, per individual, in 1900 was approximately 90 lbs annually. This was up from 18 lbs annually in 1800. In 2009, more than 50% of Americans took in 180 lbs of sugar annually. Guess what the obesity rate in was 1900? It was 3.4% [110]. Even to an untrained eye, the direct relationship is obvious.

This has lead to the low carb craze. I'll be honest, I took part in this craze in the early 2000's. I even lost some weight. But what does the science say about "low carb" diets? As a physician following a low carbohydrate diet, you would have thought I knew the science behind its mechanism of action–but I did not. And why have so many lost weight using a low-carb dietary plan? What is the long term impact of low carb diets? Carbohydrates have been around for along time. Why now are carbs causing such havoc in our metabolisms? My father-in-law (80), recalls eating meals very high in carbs, but rare in simple sugars. Recent generations are not the first to be exposed to sugar. Likely, the extreme volumes of simple sugars documented above are the culprit.

The science on low carb diets in the short term is good. Eric C. Westman did a very thorough review of the literature on low carbohydrate diets from 1966 to 1999 [111]. Thirty-two articles were included

---

109  Flegal KM, Carroll MD, Ogden CL, Johnson CL. Prevalence and trends in obesity among US adults, 1999-2000. JAMA. 2002;288:1723-7.

110  Mercola J. This Addictive commonly used food feeds cancer cells, triggers weight gain, and promotes premature aging. Mercola.com. Apr 20 2010.

111  Westman EC. A review of very low carbohydrate diets for weight loss. J Clin Outcomes Manage. Jul/Aug 1999;6(7):36-40.

in the analysis. The results of his meta-analysis found that low carbohydrate diets (defined as 40 grams daily) did result in statistically significant weight loss. Short term weight loss 10 lbs was found in 6 studies [112] [113] [114] [115] [116] [117]. But many of the low carb dieters were found to be restricting calories as well. So, which is it–the low carb diet or calorie restriction. Three additional studies, however, showed that statistically significant short-term weight loss in low carb diets does occur in the absence of calorie restriction [20] [23] [118]. Many think like I use too–low carbohydrate diets result in weight loss due to concomitant calorie restriction, but here the science shows that is simply not the case. The 3 studies listed above help to put that too rest. Low carbohydrate diets ( 40 grams) do result in weight loss independent from calorie restriction. The average weight loss in the groups were 10 lbs per month. That is pretty nice weight loss.

How do low carb diets work? Low carbohydrate diets decrease appetite, improve insulin sensitivity, improve blood glucose control, lower HgbA1C, lower triglyceride, and lower cholesterol levels [33]. Calorie intake did decrease from 3111 kcal/day to 2164 kcal/day in

112  Larosa JC, Fry AG, Muesing R, Rosing DR. Effects of high-protein, low-carbohydrate dieting on plasma lipoproteins and body weight. J Am Diet Assoc. 1980;77:264-70.

113  Golay A et al. Similar weight loss with low- or high-carbohydrate diets. Am J Clin Nutr. 1996;63:174-8.

114  Willi SM et al. The effects of a high-protein, low-fat, ketogenic diet on adolescents with morbid obesity: body composition, blood chemistries, and sleep abnormalities. Pediatrics. 1998;101:61-7.

115  Young CM, Scanlan SS, Im HS, Lutwak L. Effect of body composition and other parameters in obese young men of carbohydrate level of reduction diet. Am J Clin Nutr. 1971;24:290-6.

116  Rabast U, Vornberger, KH, Ehl M. Loss of weight, sodium and water in obese persons consuming a high- or low-carbohydrate diet. Ann Nutr Metab. 1981;25:341-9.

117  Rickman F, Mitchell N, Dingman J, Dalen JE. Changes in serum cholesterol during the Stillman diet. JAMA. 1974;228:54-8.

118  Worthington BS, Taylor LE. Balanced low-calorie vs high-protein-low-carbohydrate reducing diets. I. Weight loss, nutrient intake, and subjective evaluation. J Am Diet Assoc. 1974;64:47-51.

this study. That only makes sense, if carbs make up such a large part of the American diet today, a reduction in carb intake will result in some decrease in calorie intake—whether or not it is significant. This is not a contradiction of the above paragraph, just simple logic.

Short-term dietary carbohydrate restriction clearly has health benefits. Particular health benefits are found in lipid metabolism, insulin resistance, and weight loss. The question is what are the long term effects of a low carbohydrate lifestyle and is a low carbohydrate diet something that everyone should incorporate? There are limited studies present to answer these questions. But what studies are present, have shown some potential ominous signs. Long-term carbohydrate restriction has been associated with heart arrhythmias, heart contractile dysfunction, sudden death, kidney damage, and cancer to name a few [119]. What did the people in these studies increase to replace the decrease in carbohydrates? There are to many variables left unanswered. The lack of good, solid long-term data on long-term carbohydrate diets limits the recommendation for that here. But, the evidence clearly favors a reduction in overall carbohydrate intake in those eating a typical American diet, those that are overweight, those with insulin resistance, and those with abnormal lipids. Of course, this includes a lot of people these days (at least, approximately 67% of Americans today). The point is, some dietary carbohydrate reduction is beneficial to most people, however the severe carbohydrate restriction found in many of the popular diets today have limited use long-term and are likely only beneficial in the short-term through an induction phase of weight loss.

There is definite scientific support for a variant of the low carb diet in cancer. This variant of the low carb diet is called the ketogenic diet. Specifically, a ketogenic diet replaces the dietary carbohydrate intake with an increase in the fat intake in the diet. Cancer loves sugar!

119 Bilsborough SA, Crow TC. Low-carbohydrate diets: what are the potential short- and long-term health implications? Asia Pac J Clin Nutr. 2003;12(4):396-404.

Cancer primarily uses glucose as its source of Energy. By eliminating sugar in the diet and increasing fat in the diet, the adaptable healthy cells are preferentially selected to use fats as the primary source of energy while cancer cells are selected to starve through the elimination of glucose. A ketogenic diet has been shown to use the inflexible metabolism of the cancer cells against itself. A ketogenic diet has been shown to be useful in many different cancers: brain, colon, lung, and breast [120] [121] [122] [123] [124].

Many would say that cancer cells have evolved to metabolic superiority compared to healthy cells. That could not be further from the truth. Cancer cells have evolved to rely solely on a limited metabolism called substrate-level metabolism. Healthy, efficient energy metabolism is called oxidative phosphorylation. Oxidative phosphorylation is the pathway preferentially used by healthy cells. In contrast, substrate-level metabolism is an inefficient energy production process dependent primarily on glucose. This is known as the Warburg effect [125] [126] [127] [128] [129]. Nearly all cancers, irregardless of

---

120  Lopez-Rios F et al. Loss of the mitochondrial bioenergetic capacity underlies the glucose avidity of carcinomas. Cancer Res. Oct 1 2007;67(19):9013-9017.

121  Cuezva JM et al. The bioenergetic signature of cancer: a marker of tumor progression. Cancer Res. 2002;62:6674-81.

122  Isidoro A et al. Breast carcinomas fulfill the Warburg hypothesis and provide metabolic markers of cancer prognosis. Carcinogenesis. 2005;26:2095-104.

123  Cuezva JM et al. The bioenergetic signature of lung adenocarcinomas is a molecular marker of cancer diagnosis and prognosis. Carcinogenesis. 2004;25:1157-63.

124  Seyfried TN. Metabolic management of brain cancer. Biochimica et Biophysica Acta (BBA)-Bioenergetics. June 2011;1807(6):577-594.

125  Seyfried TN, Mukherjee P. Targeting energy metabolism in brain cancer: review and hypothesis. Nutr Metab (Lond) 2005, 2:30.

126  Semenza GL et al. The metabolism of tumours': 70 years later. Novartis Found Symp 2001;240:251-260, discussion:260-264.

127  Ristow M. Oxidative metabolism in cancer growth. Curr Opin Clin Nutr Metab Care. 2006;9:339-345.

128  Gatenby RA, Gillies RJ. Why do cancers have high aerobic glycolysis? Nat Rev Cancer. 2004;4:891-899.

129  Gogvadze V, Orrenius S, Zhivotovsky B. Mitochondria in cancer cells: what is so special about them? Trends Cell Biol. 2008;18:165-173.

origin, utilize this form of cellular metabolism. This substrate-level phosphorylation can also be driven by amino acids–particularly glutamine [130] [131] [132]. In contrast, healthy cells have the biological advantage. Healthy cells can adapt their cellular machinery to make energy from many sources, including fats through ketosis.

That is what the science says on carbohydrates.

What about fat? We must get over the idea that dietary fat intake equals body fat accumulation. Scientifically speaking, this is just not the case. That would be like saying that dietary intake of cholesterol is the cause of high blood cholesterol. That is what marketing portrays, but it simply is not true. It doesn't matter what marketing says, all that matters is physiology.

It is about the fat quality. All fats are not created equally. There are polynsaturated fats, there are monosaturated fats, there are saturated fats, and there are trans fats. The more detrimental fats are the saturated fats, but particularly the trans fats are the worst. Total fat intake has declined over the past 30 years (thanks to the low fat craze). In comparison, the saturated and trans fats have declined less than the total fat intake decline [133]. So, though fat intake has declined slightly, the percentage of "bad" fats have increased.

If fat intake was the driving force behind obesity and poor health, then the recent decline in fat intake would benefit both–but it has not. **The obesity rate has actually shown an inverse rise with the advent of the "low fat" diet** [134]. In fact, increase intake of certain fats,

130  Yuneva M. Finding an "Achilles' heel" of cancer: the role of glucose and glutamine metabolism in the survival of transformed cells. Cell Cycle. 2008;7:2083-2089.

131  Deberardinis RJ, Cheng T. Q's next: the diverse functions of glutamine in metabolism, cell biology and cancer. Oncogene. 2009.

132  Yang C et al. Glioblastoma cells require glutamate dehydrogenase to survive impairments of glucose metabolism or Akt signaling. Cancer Res. 2009.

133  Lichtenstein AH et al. Nutr Rev. May 1998;56(5 Pt 2):S3-19.

134  Heini AF, Weinsier RL. Divergent trends in obesity and fat intake patterns: the American paradox. Am J Med. Mar 1997;102(3):259-64.

omega-3 [135] [136] and coconut oil [137] [138], have been shown to aid weight loss and thus improve health. Chew on that for a moment. This is often a difficult concept for many to overcome. An increase in certain fats can cause weight loss. Fat equals weight loss? Wow! Again, it is about the quality of the fat and then the quantity of that quality.

I would be derelict in my duties if I didn't mention a recent study that found an increased risk of aggressive prostate cancer in men with the highest levels of omega-3 in blood. This study is everything that is wrong with medicine today (remember the politicization of medicine). The meta-analysis found a 71% increased risk of prostate cancer in those with the highest levels of the essential fatty acids ALA, DHA and EPA [139]. Though a reduction in risk was found in DPA. The conclusion of a publication on this article says it all: "the researchers could not be certain whether the study's participants ate oily fish or took omega-3 supplements...". What?! The analysis occurred over a 7 year time frame. The levels of omega-3 were determined at the beginning of the study. No follow up analysis of omega-3 levels were obtained over the 7 years of the analysis. This study did not look at a group of men taking omega-3 supplements and compare them to a group of men not taking omega 3 supplements. This study couldn't even note if this was from omega-3 supplements, from fish intake, or from lipid

---

135   Golub N, Geba D, Mousa SA, Williams G, Block RC. Greasing the wheels of managing overweight and obesity with omega-3 fatty acids. Med Hypotheses. Dec 2011;77(6):1114-20.

136   Li JJ, Huang CJ, Xie D. Anti-obesity effects of conjugated linoleic acid, docosahexaenoic acid, and eicosapentaenoic acid. Mol Nutr Food Res. Jun 2008;52(6):631-45.

137   Liau KM, Lee YY, Chen CK, Rasool AHG. An open-label pilot study to assess the efficacy and safety of virgin coconut oil in reducing visceral adiposity. ISRN Pharmacol. 2011;2011:949686.

138   Assuncao ML, Ferreira HS, dos Santos AF, Cabral CR Jr, Florencio TM. Effects of dietary coconut oil on the biochemical and anthropmetric profiles of women presenting abdominal obesity. Lipids. Jul 2009;44(7):593-601.

139   Sorongon-Legaspi MK et al. Blood level omega-3 fatty acids as risk determinant molecular biomarker for prostate cancer. Prostate Cancer. 2013:875615.

metabolism. This study just looked at those with prostate cancer and then evaluated their blood omega-3 levels.

This study in question did not look at the saturated fats levels. This study did not look at the trans-fat levels. This study did not look at glucose metabolism. This study did not look at inflammatory cytokines. Were these individuals taking supplements prior to the diagnosis of cancer? Did these individuals change their diets to a healthier diet once diagnosed with cancer? What dietary changes, if any, were recommended? Why did the authors change the variables of the study that they looked at in the meta-analysis? These are just a few simple questions not answered. One cannot cherry pick data from a study designed to look at its effect on A, then look at X. That is like taking a test and then trying to change the answers after the test has already been graded. The leap in association made here is as big as jumping across the grand canyon with a pogo stick.

The conclusion of the authors is that men should limit their fish intake to 1-2 meals per week. The only problem with that is the inuit eskimos. The inuit eskimos eat 8 grams of omega-3 a day. Their diet is mainly fat and protein from fish, seal, and walrus. They are heavy smokers, as society goes, yet they have low cardiovascular disease and the inuit eskimoe men have low levels of prostate cancer [140]. However, recently the inuits have undergone a change to a more western style diet high in carbohydrates. The result has been an increase in breast, prostate, colon, and lung cancer rates [141].

This study flies in the face of the evidence of the ketogenic diet and in the knowledge of cancer metabolism (discussed above). As described above, cancer uses glucose as it primary energy source.

---

140  Dewailly E et al. Inuit are protected against prostate cancer. Cancer Epidemiol Biomarkers Prev. Sep 2003;12(9):926-7.

141  Friborg JT, Melbye M. Cancer patterns in Inuit populations. The Lancet Oncology. 2008;9:892-900.

The ketogenic diet uses a high fat diet to preferentially select healthy cell metabolism from dysfunctional cancer cell metabolism.

What does the scientific evidence say about omega-3's? Omega-3 intake has been shown to reduce inflammation [142] [143] [144] [145], improve insulin resistance [146], improve the parameters of metabolic syndrome [147] [148] [149], slow/inhibit cancer growth [150] [151] [152] [153] [154] [155], inhibit

142 Calder PC. n-3 Polyunsaturated fatty acids, inflammation, and inflammatory diseases. Am J Clin Nutr. June 2006;83(6):S1505-1519S.

143 Endres S et al. The effect of dietary supplementation with n-3 polyunsaturated fatty acids on the synthesis of Interleukin-1 and Tumor Necrosis Factor by mononuclear cells. N Engl J Med. 1989;320:265-271.

144 Rose, D. P. Connolly, J. M. (2000) Regulation of tumor angiogenesis by dietary fatty acids and eicosanoids. Nutr. Cancer 37:119-127.

145 Yang, P., Felix, E., Madden, T., Chan, D. Newman, R. A. (2002) Relative formation of PGE2 and PGE3 by eicosapentaenoic acid (EPA) and docosahexaenoic acid (DHA) in human lung cancer cells. Proc. Am. Assoc. Cancer Res. 43 number 1533 (abs.).

146 Da Young O et al. GPR120 is an omega-3 fatty acid receptor mediating potent anti-inflammatory and insulin-sensitizing effects. Cell. Sept 3 2010;142(5):687-698.

147 Agrawal R, Gomez-Pinilla F. 'Metabolic syndrome' in the brain: deficiency in omega-3 fatty acid exacerbates dysfunctions in insulin receptor signalling and cognition. J Physiology. May 15 2012;590:2485-2499.

148 Carpentier YA, Portois L, Malaisse WJ. n-3 fatty acids and the metabolic syndrome. Am J Clin Nutr. Jun 2006;83(6 suppl):1499S-1504S.

149 Poudyal H et al. Omega-3 fatty acids and metabolic syndrome: effects and emerging mechanisms of action. Prog Lipid Res. Oct 2011;50(4):372-87.

150 Begin, M. E., Ells, G., Das, U. N. Horrobin. D. F. (1986) Differential killing of human carcinoma cells supplemented with n-3 and n-6 polyunsaturated fatty acids. J. Natl. Cancer Inst. 77:1053-1062.

151 Deschner, E. E., Lytle, J. S., Wong, G., Ruperto, J. F. Newmark, H. L. (1990) The effect of dietary omega-3 fatty acids (fish oil) on azoxymethanol-induced focal areas of dysplasia and colon tumor incidence. *Cancer* **66**:2350-2356.

152 Fernandes, G., Friedrichs, W., Schultz, J. Venkatraman, J. (1989) Modulation of MCF-7 tumor cell growth in nude mice by omega-3 fatty acid diet. Breast Cancer Res. Treat. 14:179 (abs.).

153 Reddy, B. S. Sugie, S. (1988) Effect of different levels of omega-3 and omega-6 fatty acids on azoxymethane-induced colon carcinogenesis in F344 rats. Cancer Res. 48:6642-6647.

154 Rose, D. P. Connolly, J. M. (1993) Effects of dietary omega-3 fatty acids on human breast cancer growth and metastasis in nude mice. J. Natl. Cancer Inst. 85:1743-1747.

155 Connolly, J. M., Coleman, M. Rose, D. P. (1997) Effects of dietary fatty acids on DU145 human prostate cancer cell growth in athymic nude mice. Nutr. Cancer 29:114-119.

oncogene activation [156] [157], inhibit angiogenesis (new blood vessel growth required by cancer) [158] [159] [160] [161], and reduce weight [162] [163] [164]. All of these parameters will improve health and reduce cancer risk.

And then there is Protein? Protein, protein, and more protein has been the answer for a lot of dieters recently. I see clients that will use diet programs that require 4-5 protein shakes daily. Almost an exclusive protein diet. More like a ketogenic diet without the fats–not very healthy. Many confuse high protein diets with low-carb diets. They are not the same. Several studies have shown that low carb diets don't translate to high protein intake [165] [166]. Common low-carb diets are the

156  Collett, E. D., Davidson, L. A., Fan, Y.-Y., Lupton, J. R. Chapkin, R. S. (2001) n-6 and n-3 polyunsaturated fatty acids differentially modulate oncogenic Ras activation in colonocytes. Am. J. Physiol. Cell Physiol. 280:C1066-C1075.

157  Liu, G., Bibus, D. M., Bode, A. M., Ma, W.-Y., Holman, R. T. Dong, Z. (2001) Omega 3 but not omega 6 fatty acids inhibit AP-1 activity and cell transformation in JB6 cells. Proc. Natl. Acad. Sci. U.S.A. 98:7510-7515.

158  Bing, R. J., Miyataka, M., Rich, K. A., Hanson, N., Wang, X., Slosser, H. D. Shi, S.-R. (2001) Nitric oxide, prostanoids, cyclooxygenase, and angiogenesis in colon and breast cancer. Clin. Cancer Res. 7:3385-3392.

159  Form, D. M. Auerbach, R. (1983) PGE$_2$ and angiogenesis. Proc. Soc. Exp. Biol. Med. 172:214-218.

160  McCarty, M. F. (1996) Fish oil may impede tumour angiogenesis and invasiveness by down-regulating protein kinase C and modulating eicosanoid production. Med. Hypotheses 46:107-115.

161  Wen, B., Deutsch, E., Opolon, P., Auperin, A., Frascogna, V., Connault, E. Bourhis, J. (2003) n-3 polyunsatyrated fatty acids decrease mucosal/epidermal reactions and enhance antitumour effect of ionising radiation with inhibition of tumour angiogenesis. Br. J. Cancer 89:1102-1107.

162  Flock MR et al. Immunometabolic role of long-chain omega-3 fatty acids in obesity-induced inflammation. Diabetes Metab Res Rev. Apr 16 2013. doi:10.1002/dmrr.2414.

163  Buckley JD, Howe PR. Anti-obesity effects of long-chain omega-3 polyunsaturated fatty acids. Obes Rev. Nov 2009;10(6):648-59.

164  Lorente-Cebrian S et al. Role of omega-3 fatty acids in obesity, metabolic syndrome, and cardiovascular diseases: a review of the evidence. J Physiol Biochem. June 22 2013.

165  Westman EC, Yancy WS, Edman JS, Tomlin KF, Perkins CE. Effect of 6-month adherence to a very low carbohydrate diet program. The American Journal of Medicine. Jul 2002;113(1):30-36.

166  Boden G, Sargrad K, Homko C, Mozzoli M, Stein TP. Effect of a low-carbohydrate diet on appetite, blood glucose levels, and insulin resistance in obese patients with type 2 diabetes. Ann Intern Med. Mar 2005;142(6):403-11.

Atkins and South Beach diets. These may or may not include high protein, as a lot these diets have significant fat content. A lot of the fat content turns out to be the saturated and trans fat variety–bad fat.

High protein intake has long been used by athletes to maximize performance and enhance recovery. The first reported use of protein supplements was by the German team in the XI Olympics in Berlin [167]. This has translated into amino acid supplementation ranking in the top 5 of supplements used by athletes today [168].

Studies on improved performance with protein supplementation are mixed. Most studies do not find benefit in increased muscle mass or muscle performance in the non-athlete [169] [170] [171]. A 1999 review of the current available data at the time, found no benefit in athletic performance from protein supplementation. There was some limited evidence that certain amino acids favored an anabolic state (building and regenerative phase), but found no contribution to improved athletic performance [172].

Contrast these conclusions with the concept that each individual is different. A non-athlete just starting a 20-30 minute exercise program is unlikely to need or benefit from additional protein supplementation. In contrast, an athlete's needs are quite different.

---

167  Schenk P. Die Verpflegung von 4700 wettkampfern aus 42 Nationen im Olympischen Dorf wahrend der XI. Olympischen Spiel 1936 zu Berlin. Muench Med Wochenschr. 1936.83:1535-1539.

168  Lawrence M, Kirby D. Nutrition and sports supplements: Fact or fiction. Journal of Clinical Gastroenterology. 2002;35:299-306.

169  Hoffman JR et al. Effects of protein supplementation on muscular performance and resting hormonal changes in college football players. Journal of Sports Science and Medicine. 2007;6:85-92.

170  Candow DG et al. Protein supplementation before and after resistance training in older men. European Journal of Applied Physiology. 2006a;97:548-556.

171  Candow et al. Effect of whey and soy protein supplementation combined with resistance training in young adults. International Journal of Sport Nutrition and Exercise Metabolism. 2006b;16:233-244.

172  Kreider RB. Effects of protein and amino-acid supplementation on athletic performance. Sports Science. 1999;3(1).

An athlete undergoing extensive training experiences continuous muscle breakdown and ongoing muscle repair and may benefit from additional protein. It is easy to see that extra support for repair is required to meet the high demand for muscle damage and repair in the athlete versus the non-athlete [173] [174] [175]. In the athlete, a positive nitrogen balance through amino acid supplementation can provide improved repair, quicker muscle recovery, and thus improved performance [176].

The discrepancy in benefit may be due to the different amino acids used in the athlete and the non-athlete. The different amino acids are absorbed differently and this can effect the biological availability. Amino acids are not created equally–nor are they absorbed the same. In fact, only casein and low, repetitive dosing of whey protein have been shown to favor protein balance (as measure by leucine levels). The benefit of amino acid supplementation with training probably occurs primarily through improved muscle recovery (as stated above). In fact, studies have shown that amino acid intake immediately surrounding exercise, significantly improved protein synthesis with a concomitant decrease in protein breakdown [177] [178] [179]. This would obviously favor muscle recovery. Recovery

173   Tipton KD et al. Ingestion of casein and whey proteins result in muscle anabolism after resistance exercise. Medicine Science in Sports Exercise. 2004;36:2073-2081.

174   Lemon PWR et al. Protein requirements and muscle mass/strength changes during intensive training in novice bodybuilders. Journal of Applied Physiology. 1992;73:767-775.

175   Tarnopolsky MA et al. Evaluation of protein requirements for trained strength athletes. Journal of Applied Physiology. 1992;73:1986-1995.

176   Kraemer WJ et al. The effects of amino acid supplementaitonon hormonal responses to overreaching. Metabolism. 2006;55:282-291.

177   Bilsborough S, Mann N. A review of issues of dietary protein intake in humans. Int J Sport Nutr Exer Metab. 2006/16:129-152.

178   Dangin M et al. The digestion rate of protein is an independent regulating factor of postprandial protein retention. Am J Physiol Endocrinol Metab. 2001;280:E340-E348.

179   Forslund AH et al. Effect of protein intake and physical activity on 24-h pattern and rate of macronutrient utilization. Am J Physiol. 1999;276:E964-E976.

is extremely important in any intense training or athletic performance. One cannot discount the benefit of an improved recovery phase in training and athletic events or simply in a exercise program. One can even see logically how improved recovery could lead to reduced injury and improved performance, whatever the goal may be. Though studies have not consistently found this.

Final answer on Amino acids? Amino acids are beneficial in the recovery phase of exercise–especially in the athlete. Amino acid replacement in the first 2 hours after training helps to quickly restore muscle glycogen stores, end the muscle breakdown (catabolic phase) and restore muscle healing (anabolic phase) [180]. This is extremely important in the highly trained athlete–especially the athlete that competes multiple times a day or in successive days. The quicker the recovery, the shorter the interval to a repeat and improved athletic performance.

Numerous studies have shown that the Testosterone to Cortisol ratio (T:C) decreases during training and increases during the recovery phase. Translation–Cortisol is catabolic and Testosterone is anabolic. This reveals the catabolic phase of training and the anabolic phase of recovery. What is interesting is that dietary protein intake has been shown to be associated with an increase in basal Testosterone production [181]. This increased basal Testosterone production could reduce the catabolic phase of training, increase the anabolic phase of recovery, increase recovery through a shortened recovery time, improve muscle growth, increase Testosterone production, and increase performance. Everything a man should want, whether he is a professional athlete or a weekend exercise warrior.

---

180 Ivy JL. Regulation of muscle glycogen repletion, muscle protein synthesis and repair following exercise. J Sports Science Medicine;2004(3):131-138.

181 Volek JS et al. Testosterone and cortisol in relationship to dietary nutrients and resistance exercise. Journal of Applied Physiology. Jan 1997;82(1):49-54.

For the athlete and the non-athlete, increased basal Testosterone production will increase muscle growth. Muscle is concentrated with mitochondria which are the energy factories of the cell. Increased capacity to make energy will increase the energy balance of the individual and reduce stored energy (i.e., fat loss).

How does this apply to those not in training, or competing in athletic events, or the just non-athletic? The ability to provide a nutritional environment that favors lean body mass and aids recovery with any exercise will only help lead to health. I see many middle-aged and older men struggle with declining muscle mass. A man with declining muscle mass has a reduced capacity to create energy and burn excess fat. The result is a severe energy imbalance—a negative energy balance. Any organism with a negative energy balance will not perform well or live long.

In contrast to the inconsistent findings with performance, there appear to be many advantages to increasing protein in your diet. Higher protein intake has been shown to be thermogenic [182], reduces appetite [183], aid weight loss [184], improves lipid metabolism [185], preserves lean body mass (muscle) [186], and improves insulin resistance [187]. Branched chain amino acids are a common

---

182  Johnston C, Day C, Swan P. Postprandial thermogenesis is increased 100% on a high protein, low-fat diet versus a high carbohydrate, low-fat diet in healthy young women. J Am Coll Nutr. 2002;21:55-61.

183  Stubbs RJ. Nutrition Society Medal Lecture. Appetite, feeding behaviour and energy balance in human subjects. Proc Nutr Soc. 1998;57:341-356.

184  Cordain L, Eaton SB, Miller JB, Mann N, Hill K. The paradoxical nature of hunter-gatherer diets: meat based yet non-atherogenic. Eur J Clin Nutr. 2002;56:S42-S52.

185  Wolfe BM, Piche LA. Replacement of carbohydrate by protein in a conventional fat diet reduces cholesterol and triglyceride concentrations in healthy normolipidemic subjects. Clin Invest Med. 1999;22:140-148.

186  Layman DK, Shiue H, Sather C, Erickson DJ, Baum J. Increased dietary protein modifies glucose and insulin homeostasis in adult woman during weight loss. J Nutr. 2003;133:405-410.

187  Piatti P et al. Hypercaloric high protein diets improve glucose oxidation and spares lean body mass: comparison to hypocaloric high carbohydrate diet. Metabolism. 1994;43:1481-1487.

type of amino acid used by athletes today. A recent study found that branched chain amino acid levels were positively associated with improvement in insulin resistance and weight loss [188]. The more branched chain amino acids, the better the insulin sensitivity and the lower the weight.

Inflammation and diet?

Nutrition is more than macronutrients and micronutrients. Nutrition is more than just calories in and calories out. Improper nutrition can be the source of inflammation and inflammation is a pre-requisite for disease. Proper nutrition can be the beginning of health and improper nutrition can be the beginning of disease.

In chapter 12 I talk about how inflammation arising from the gut, in the form of dysbiosis (imbalance of the gut bacteria), can cause type II Diabetes. Here, I am simply talking about inflammation from the foods that we eat. In many individuals, inflammation begins the moment they open their mouth–"out of the mouth, the heart speaks". With regards to inflammatory foods, into the mouth, the body is.

We are all familiar with the idea that foods high in sugar and trans fats are bad for us. But, what if foods themselves were the source of inflammation. These foods can be of the supposably good, healthy variety like broccoli and cauliflower. However, if the immune system reacts to the presence of even good, healthy foods, then they can be the cause inflammation and that is unhealthy. When it comes to foods, inflammation can be a equal opportunity offender. Inflammation can be the result of both healthy and/or unhealthy foods. Just because food is healthy, like cruciferous vegetables, does not mean that they cannot cause inflammation and thus be unhealthy for some.

---

188  Shah SH et al. Branched-chain amino acid levels are associated with improvement in insulin resistance with weight loss. Diabetologia. Feb 2012;55(2):321-30.

How does this happen?

There are many factors that contribute to food sensitivities: processed foods, chronic antibiotics, dysbiosis, and genetically modified foods (GMO). The end result is a leaky gut. The term "leaky gut" does not imply diarrhea, but actually the opposite. Undigested food particles "leak" from the gut into the body. The constant insult on the gut lining leads to it's break down. The gut lining is one cell thick with tight junctions. When these tight junctions begin to break down, food particles break through and the immune system reacts. Essentially, the immune system thinks it is being attacked by that food particle. Who would have thought that the body can think it is being attacked by romaine lettuce, but that is a simple summary how food sensitivities can develop.

Another example is Celiac disease. Celiac disease is an auto-immune disease precipitated by the adaptive immune system in response to gluten. In celiac disease, antibodies are produced that attack the lining of the gut, particularly the villi, of the small intestine that results in small intestine damage and malabsorption.

What I am talking about here are food sensitivities. Food sensitivities will not have the immediate reactions seen with peanut allergies or Celiac disease. But, they will present with more indolent, delayed symptoms, often mistaken for other causes. These food sensitivities are not genetic, but rather unique to the individual and the result of the gut environment. The symptoms can range from bloating, to headaches, to even rashes, and the non-discrete brain fog. These symptoms can occur immediately, but the vast majority will occur hours to even days later. This delay in symptom presentation can leave the individual and the medical provider puzzled as to the cause.

My daughter is the perfect example of a person suffering with a food sensitivity reaction. My daughter was having problems with rosacea. She did not like it. Traditional medical dogma called for chronic antibiotic therapy. We decided to test her for food sensitivities. Turns out, her rosacea was due to a food sensitivity to dairy products. Now, as long as she avoids dairy products, there is no rosacea. Her inflammatory response to dairy products was manifesting in her cheeks as rosacea. We were able to provide a simple, customized, solutions-based therapy for my daughter through the elimination of an identified food sensitivity. No antibiotics required.

Only recently, physicians and providers that used the term food sensitivity were ridiculed and ostracized. However, the 2011 International Celiac Disease symposium in Oslo, Norway brought gluten sensitivity to the forefront in medicine. The 2011 symposium was the first to define and recognize gluten sensitivity as a distinct separate pathological process. Both gluten sensitivity and celiac disease involve immune reactions to gluten. The 2011 symposium defined gluten sensitivity as a separate immune response, distinct from that found in celiac disease. Gluten sensitivity is a response of the innate immune system to gluten. Gluten sensitivity lacks the characteristics of the adaptive immune response (antibodies) and intestinal damage found in celiac disease, but presents with extra-intestinal symptoms through non-antibody mediated signaling [189].

Inflammation doesn't end with food sensitivities. Inflammation can also occur from the balance of foods that we eat. The perfect example here can be found in the balance of the fats that we Americans eat. There are many different kids of fats, also known as essential fatty acids: omega-3's,

---

189  ICDS. 14th International Coeliac Disease Symposium 2011. June 20-22 2011. Oslo, Norway.

omega-6's, omega 9's, saturated fats, and trans fats. Dr. Floyd H Chilton describes this in his book *Inflammation* Nation [190]. A good healthy balance of omega-3 to omega-6 would be in the range of 1:3. However, the typical American diet is in a ratio of 1:24. Omega-3 are commonly found in the "fish oils" that are so often discussed. Omega-3's have many benefits, one of which is their anti-inflammatory effects. Studies have consistently shown that EPA and DHA are the two most important omega-3's. In contrast, the omega-6's, such as the like of arachadonic acid, tend to be very pro-inflammatory. Common sources of omega-6's are seeds, seed oil, nuts, corn, primrose oil, and borage oil. Our bodies need omega-6's, just not in the disproportionate imbalance one finds in the typical processed American diet. That is the point of Dr. Chilton–our nation is a nation of inflammation, simply because the fats in our diet are out of balance.

Lets take one step deeper. What is the link between over-nutrition and obesity? If your answer is excess calories, then you would be correct. However, the mechanism of action is inflammation. Inflammation is the result of the over-nutrition. Excess calories are causing the inflammation that results in obesity. Dietary induced obesity (DIO) is the result of inflammation [191]. Stated differently: over-nutrition causes inflammation that results in obesity. The statement, "obesity is simply calories in and calories out", is devoid of solutions.

---

190   Chilton FH. Inflammation Nation: The first clinically proven eating plan to end our Nation's secret epidemic. FIRESIDE. New York NY. 2005.

191   Cai D, Liu T. Inflammatory cause of metabolic syndrome via brain stress and NF-kappaB. Aging (Albany NY). Feb 2012;4(2):98-115.

Inflammation leads to insulin resistance [192] [193] [194], metabolic syndrome [195] [196], type II diabetes [197] [198], cardiovascular disease [199] [200] [201], neurodegenerative disease [202] [203], and cancer [204] [205]. Science has shown that inflammation causes central dysfunction of the hypothalamus [206] [207] and peripheral dysfunction of the GLUT4 receptor. The peripheral dysfunction of the GLUT4 receptor is responsible

192  Shoelson SE, Lee Jongsoon, Goldfine AB. Inflammation and insulin resistance. J Clin Invest. 2006;116(7):1793-1801.

193  Petersen KF, Shulman GI. Etiology of insulin resistance. Am. J. Med. 2006;119:S10–S16.

194  Schenk S, Saberi M, Olefsky JM. Insulin sensitivity: modulation by nutrients and inflammation. J. Clin. Invest. 2008;118:2992–3002.

195  Lehrke M, Lazar MA. Inflamed about obesity. Nat. Med. 2004;10:126–7.

196  Ferrante AW., Jr Obesity-induced inflammation: a metabolic dialogue in the language of inflammation. J. Intern. Med. 2007;262:408–14.

197  Lowell BB, Shulman GI. Mitochondrial dysfunction and type 2 diabetes. Science. 2005;307:384–7.

198  Petersen KF, Befroy D, Dufour S, Dziura J, Ariyan C, Rothman DL, DiPietro L, Cline GW, Shulman GI. Mitochondrial dysfunction in the elderly: possible role in insulin resistance. Science. 2003;300:1140–2.

199  Bernal-Mizrachi C, Gates AC, Weng S, Imamura T, Knutsen RH, DeSantis P, Coleman T, Townsend RR, Muglia LJ, Semenkovich CF. Vascular respiratory uncoupling increases blood pressure and atherosclerosis. Nature. 2005;435:502–6.

200  Ren J, Pulakat L, Whaley-Connell A, Sowers JR. Mitochondrial biogenesis in the metabolic syndrome and cardiovascular disease. J. Mol. Med. (Berl.) 2010;88:993–1001.

201  Wisloff U, Najjar SM, Ellingsen O, Haram PM, Swoap S, Al-Share Q, Fernstrom M, Rezaei K, Lee SJ, Koch LG, et al. Cardiovascular risk factors emerge after artificial selection for low aerobic capacity. Science. 2005;307:418–20.

202  Lin MT, Beal MF. Mitochondrial dysfunction and oxidative stress in neurodegenerative diseases. Nature. 2006;443:787–95.

203  DiMauro S, Schon EA. Mitochondrial disorders in the nervous system. Annu. Rev. Neurosci. 2008;31:91–123.

204  Giovannucci E, Michaud D. The role of obesity and related metabolic disturbances in cancers of the colon, prostate, and pancreas. Gastroenterology. 2007;132:2208–25.

205  Essick EE, Sam F. Oxidative stress and autophagy in cardiac disease, neurological disorders, aging and cancer. Oxid. Med. Cell Longev. 2010;3:168–77.

206  Gregor MF, Hotamisligil GS. Inflammatory mechanisms in obesity. Annu. Rev. Immunol. 2011;29:415–45.

207  Thaler JP, Schwartz MW. Minireview: Inflammation and obesity pathogenesis: the hypothalamus heats up. Endocrinology. 2010;151:4109–15.

for the dysfunction in glucose uptake and metabolism [208]. This insulin resistance increases adiposity (particularly abdominal fat). Fat increases inflammation signaling and inflammation increases aromatase activity [209]. Aromatase is the enzyme that converts Testosterone to Estrogen. Eighty percent of Estrogen production in men comes from abdominal fat aromatase activity [210]. So, inflammation increases aromatase activity (estrogen producing enzyme) and inflammation increases adiposity (belly fat). Both, increase Testosterone to Estrogen conversion in men, which will increase weight gain and inflammation (see figure 1 below). This will lead to a vicious cycle that will result in low Testosterone in men. Notice that the effect we see is low Testosterone, but the cause is inflammation and/or excess Estrogen production. The inflammation can be the result of dysbiosis, food sensitivities, and over-nutrition.

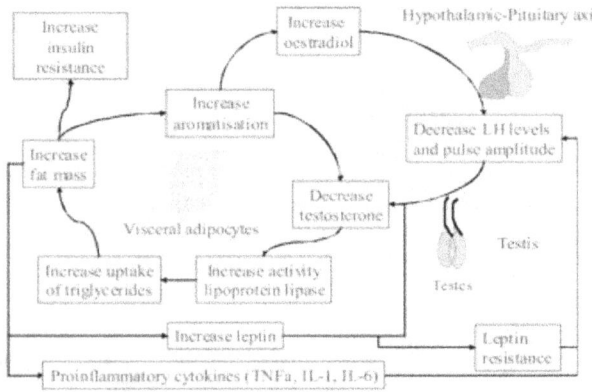

*(Figure 1 hypogonadal-obesity-adipocytokine hypothesis)* [211]

208  Armoni M, Harel C, Karnieli E. Transcriptional regulation of the GLUT4 gene: from PPAR-gamma and FOXO1 to FFA and inflammation. Trends Endocrinol Metab. Apr 2007;18(3):100-7.

209  Subbaramaiah K et al. Obesity is associated with inflammation and elevated aromatase expression in the mouse mammary gland. Cancer Prev Res (Phila). Mar 2011;4(3):329-46.

210  Kirschner MA et al. Obesity, androgens, estrogens, and cancer risk. Cancer Res;42:3281s-3285s.

211  Stanworth RD, Jones TH. Testosterone for the aging male; current evidence and recommended practice. Clin Inter Aging. March 2008;3(1):25-44.

## Xenoestrogens

You may be familiar with them. You may not. Whether or not you are, they are all around us and effect us. They are in the foods that we eat, the water that we drink, and the air that we breath. As a growing part of the environment, they are becoming a growing disruption in our physiology.

Up until recently, the effects of xenoestrogens have been ignored and those that discuss them, ridiculed. But, as the effects of the environment on our health becomes more apparent, xenoestrogens are starting to get more press. But, xenoestrogens are not new to research. Xenoestrogens have been in the research for a long time.

## What are xenoestrogens?

Xenoestrogens can be defined as environmental chemicals that mimic hormonal effects that then disrupt normal hormone function. The major hormone(s) mimicked is estrogen. It would also be safe to label xenoestrogens as environmental toxins. Anything that disrupts normal function should be labeled a toxin. But, due to the politicization of the issue, the less confrontational term used is endocrine disruptors.

Remember, the concern is with excess Estrogen, whether endogenous or exogenous, in men. Excessive Estrogen inhibits pituitary LH production, which inhibits testicular Testosterone production (see figure 2 below).

Low T results in an increased all-cause mortality rate in men. Low Testosterone and high Estrogen levels in men promotes a chronic inflammatory response. This inflammation plays a major role in just about every chronic disease associated with aging. The negative effects of xenoestrogens can be summed up in 4 effects: increased Estrogen, blocked Testosterone receptors, decrease Testosterone production through inhibition at the site of the hypothalamus and the pituitary, and increased inflammation.

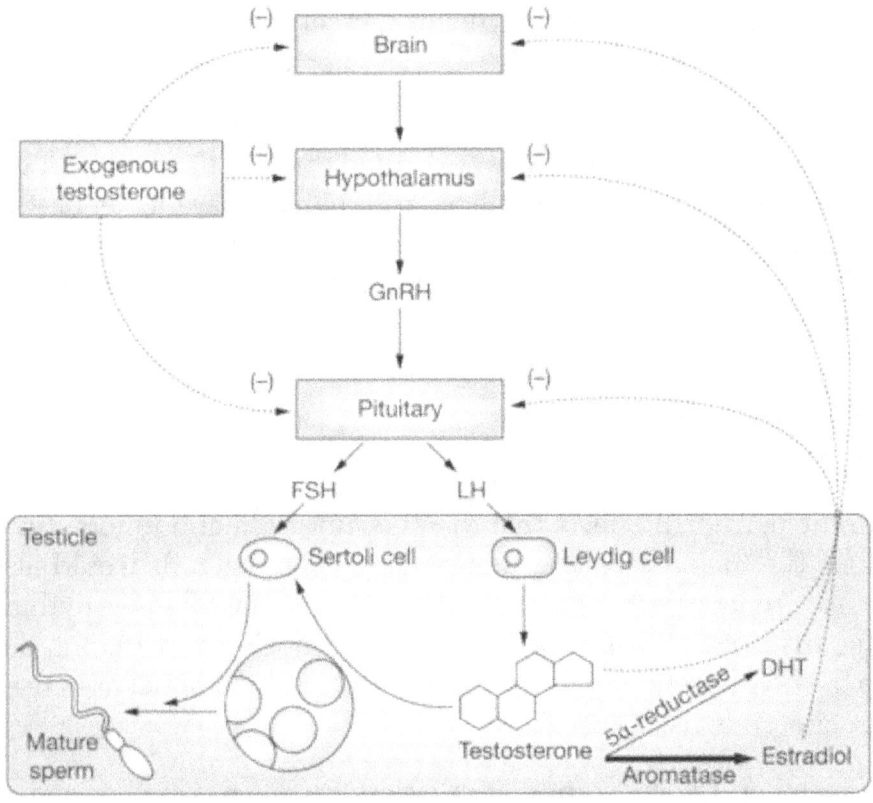

*(Figure 2 Treatment of male infertility secondary to morbid obesity )* [212]

The problem with xenoestrogens is not just their effect, but how to protect against their exposure. I discuss more about xenoestrogens in chapter 10.

212  Roth MY, Amory JK, Page ST. Treatment of male infertility secondary to morbid obesity. Nat Clin Pract Endocrinol Metab. Jul 2008;4(7):415-9.

In summary, proper nutrition lays the ground work for health or poor nutrition lays the ground work for disease. This is no more evident than in low Testosterone in men. Low Testosterone in men cannot be appropriately managed without a solid foundation on nutrition.

# CHAPTER 7

# EXERCISE

Remember, I am a recovering fat man. In 1991, I was 285 pounds. I bench pressed 425 lbs, squatted 550 lbs, had a 23 inch neck, wore size 46 pants and wore a 54 jacket.

Sure, I was a big football player, but I was also fat. I had a big tire to prove it.

Growing up, I had my fair share of exercise. I played sports. For as long as I can remember I played sports–particularly football. With that came exercise. A lot of exercise. It started when I was young, but the exercise was limited due to my young age. It wasn't until I was 13 that I started to take exercise to the extreme level. We were taught from the very beginning that more, when it comes to exercise, is the best. Nothing, I repeat nothing, was ever mentioned of recovery. This exercise regimen increased through high school. With College, came regular, heavy exercise. Whether it was off season or in season, I was lifting, running, sprinting, hitting, sweating for 2 or more hours daily. There were plenty of days that my stomach got the best of me (if you know what I mean). From sprints to heavy weight lifting, my early years were spent in extreme exercise.

Was I healthy? Good question. I am sure that there are many that would have said I was. But, in retrospect, I can tell you I was not. Sure, I could do the gasers (100 hundred yard sprints, back and forth and back and forth...you get the picture) and lift the weights. I was in shape to perform on the field, but I wasn't healthy.

One example will make my point. We opened up one season at Baylor. We were just coming out of training camp. We had just finished 3 weeks of 2-a-days and 2 weeks of regular preparation in the heat of August. August in Louisiana is HOT!!! This had followed summer training of weights and cardio, consisting of sprints, stairs, and running daily. According to most standards we were in shape. Heck, I thought I was. I remember that opening game well. If there is a hell on earth that day, it was in Waco, Texas. Half way through the 4th quarter of a very close game, I started to cramp up. I cramped up so bad, I had to come out of the game and limp to the locker room to sit in a tub of ice (thanks to a kick from Chris Bonoit, we won that game). I cramped in muscles I didn't know I had. My legs hurt for days after that. I had exercised all summer. I was healthy. Not!

I relate that old glory story to give an example of over training syndrome (OTS). We had overtrained. Don't tell my coaches that. The symptoms of that night were just the culmination of the OTS. Symptoms of OTS often go unnoticed until it is too late [213], as in my case.

Of course, there is the UTS or under training syndrome. Many know this as the couch potato syndrome. One would think this to be quit common. In my practice, I find this to be rare. When I do see a lack of exercise, it is a result of extreme fatigue, chronic pain, etc. There is not a lack of desire to exercise. They want to, they just can't. In these people, a traditional exercise regimen could actually be very detrimental due their health.

---

213  Wilmore JH, Costill DL, Kenney WL. Physiology of sport and exercise. Human Kinetics Publishers. Champaign, IL. 2008.

The majority of the people I see are already in some type of exercise regimen. In fact, the majority are considering doing more exercise because of a lack of results from the current exercise regimen. My focus on exercise comes from my experience with my patients. They do to much, they think they have to do a lot, they are told they need to do more–they overtrain.

So what is OTS? Symptoms of overtraining are the imbalance between excessive stress and lack of adequate recovery [214] [215]. Simply stated, too much exercise with too little recovery. The recovery phase of exercise is just as important as the stress phase of exercise. The stressors of life are self-evident: stressful job, deadlines, etc But, physiologic stressors (like over training) are often more dangerous because they go unrecognized. Symptoms of over training syndrome are: fatigue, depression, burnout, anxiousness, sleep pattern changes, focus changes, excessive soreness, reduce sex drive, and increased upper respiratory tract infections. But we are men. There is no such thing as over training, right? Wrong. The body can only do so much, especially when it is not supported nutritionally.

Over training syndrome is quite common in athletes [216]. Approximately 20% of elite athletes over train [217] [218]. Overtraining

214  Lehmann M, Gastmann U, Steinacker JM, Heinz N, Brouns F. Overtraining in endurance sports. A short review. Med Sport Boh Slov. 1995;4:1-6.

215  Lehmann M, Foster C, Gastmann U, Keizer HA, Steinacker JM. Definition, types, symptoms, findings, underlying mechanisms, and frequency of overtraining and overtraining syndrome. In: Overload, fatigue, performance incompetence, and regeneration in sport. New Yor: plenum 1999;1-6.

216  Bandyopadhay A, Bhattacharjee I, Sousana PK. Physiological perspective of endurance overtraining-A comprehensive update. Al Ameen J Med Sci. 2012;5(1):7-20.

217  Morgan Wp, Brown DR, Raglin JS, O'Connor PJ, Ellickson KA. Psychological monitoring of overtraining and staleness. BR J Sport Med. 1987;21:107-114.

218  Hooper SL, Mackinon LT, Gordon RD, Bachmann AW. Hormonal responses of elite swimmers to overtraining. Med Sci Sports Exerc. 1993;25:741-747.

has been documented in runners [2], swimmers [4] [5], cyclers [219], and rowers [220] [221] at high rates. No surprise, research on Olympic athletes has revealed a high prevalence of OTS [222] [223].

But, most elite athletes are aware of over training syndrome and usually have a medical team to combat OTS. However, the weekend warriors, the amateur, the "young" athlete does not. I am very concerned about the high degree of early specialization and high intensity training in young athletes today. Studies have revealed that OTS is as prevalent in the general public as in elite athletes [224] [225]. And, it is in these individuals, especially the weekend warriors and young athletes [226], that OTS goes unrecognized and serious damage can occur. In fact, it has been estimated that up to 50% of injuries are due to over training[227].

The point of the review on OTS, is that more of a good thing is not a great thing. More of a good thing can, and usually is, a

219  Kuipers H, Keizer HA. Overtraining in elite athletes: review and directions for the future. Sports Med. 1988;6:79-92.

220  Kellmann M, Gunther KD. Changes in stress and recovery in elite rowers during preparation for the Olympic Games. Medicine and Science in Sports and Exercise. 2000;32:676-683.

221  Kellmann M, Kallus KW. Recovery stress questionnaire for athletes: User manual. Human Kinetics. Champaign IL. 2001;1(suppl):70.

222  Goud Dm, Guinan D, Greenleaf C, Medbery R, Strickland M et al. Positive and negative factors influencing US Olympic athletes and coaches: Atlanta games assessment. Final grant report submitted to the US Olympic Committee, Sport Science and Technology Division, Colorado Springs. 1998.

223  Gould D, Guinan D, Greenleaf C, Medbery R, Peterson K. Factors affecting Olympic performance: Perceptions of athletes and coaches from more and less successful teams. 1999.

224  Brenner JS. Overuse injuries, overtraining, and burnout in child and adolescent athletes. American Academy of Pediatrics Council on Sports Medicine and Fitness. 2007;119:1242-1245.

225  Alves RN, Costa LOP, Samulski DM. Monitorin and prevention of overtraining in athletes. Revista Brasileira de Medicina do Esporte. 2006;12:6.

226  Maufilli N, Chan D, Aldridge M. Overuse injuries of the olecranon in young gymnasts. J Bone Joint Surg Br. 1992;74:305-308.

227  Dalton SE. Overuse injuries in adolescent athletes. Sports Med. 1992;12:58-70.

very detrimental thing for your health. In America, we love to do things to excess. Whether it be our celebrations (see Mardi Gras), our eating (see our obesity rates), or our exercise: the philosophy of Americans has been more is better and excess is great.

Just because one exercises, that does not mean the exercise is contributing to their health. That would be the same as saying eating is healthy. Well, it is if you eat the right foods, in the right balance, in the right portions. But if you eat 20 Twinkies a day, you are still eating, but not healthy. Exercise is the same. Exercise itself does not equate to health. Exercise can absolutely contribute to health, but exercise can equally be an obstacle to health.

Look back at football players again. These are highly trained, elite athletes. Yet, studies tell us that metabolic syndrome is rampant in college football players. Metabolic syndrome is the door way for many diseases. A diagnosis of Metabolic Syndrome in men requires 3 of the following 5 factors:

- Waist circumference > 40 inches
- Triglycerides ≥ 150
- HDL < 40
- blood pressure ≥ 130/85
- fasting blood glucose ≥ 110

Two studies from 2009 and 2010 revealed this. The 2009 study was done on Ohio State football players. They found that "There is a strong association between obesity and both metabolic syndrome and insulin resistance in Division 1 collegiate football players. Linemen are at significant risk for metabolic syndrome and insulin resistance compared with other positions. This may be predictive of future health problems in Division 1 collegiate football players, especially lineman" [228]. And I have seen this first hand, as two of my fellow offensive lineman that I played with have died from cardiovascular events. These events occurred in their late 20s and mid 30s.

To be fair to the Big ten, a 2010 study looked at my Tennessee Volunteers of the SEC. This study looked at the entire football team from lineman to the kickers and everyone else in between. They found that 19% of the overall players met the criteria for metabolic syndrome, 14% of the non-lineman, and 46% of the lineman met the criteria for metabolic syndrome [229]. A study published in the Journal of American College Health, looked at college football players versus non-athletes and found the metabolic syndrome rate at 46%. Their conclusions says it all, "...the increased prevalence of the metabolic syndrome and its components in the collegiate lineman may increase cardiovascular disease risk..."[230]

The NFL fairs no better. A 2008 study published by the American Journal of Cardiology found that the retired NFL lineman "exhibited a high prevalence of metabolic syndrome..." and that these levels doubled that of their non-lineman counterparts [231]. This has translated to a 52% increased risk of cardiovascular death when compared to the general population [232]. This increased risk of car-

228 Borchers JR, Clem KL, Habash DL, Nagaraja HN, Stokley LM, Best TM. Metabolic syndrome adn insulin resistance in Division 1 collegiate football players. Med Sci Spor Exer. Dec 2009;41;(12):2105-10.

229 Wilkerson GB, Bullard JT, Bartal DW. Identification of Cardiometabolic Risk among Collegiate Football Players. J Ath Train. Jan-Feb 2010;45(1):67-74.

230 Dobrosielski DA et al. Assessment of cardiovascular risk in collegiate football players and nonathletes. Journal of American College Health. Nov-Dec 2010;59(3):224-7.

231 Miller MA, Croft LB, Belanger AR, Romero-Corral A, Somers VK, Roberts AJ, Goldman ME. Prevalence of metabolic syndrome in retired National Football League players. Am J Cardiol. May 1 2008;101(9):1281-4.

232 Baron S, Rinsky R. HIOSH Mortality study of NFL football players: 1959-1988. Atlanta, GA: National Institute for Occupational Safety and Health. 1994. http://www.cdc.gov/niosh/pdfs/nflfactsheet.pdf. Accessed Nov 8, 2011.

diovascular death was found in the 1950s to the 1980s. The football players were definitely getting bigger during that stretch, but when you compare them to today's players, they look anorexic.

Most would consider college football and NFL football players to be elite athletes. They are extremely active, running, lifting weights, etc But, studies like those mentioned above reveal that these elite athletes are anything but healthy.

I have used football as an example, because of my long time experience in the sport. Of course, a lot of football players don't look like marathon runners, cyclists, or triathletes. Myself included, But, what if I told you there is mounting evidence that they may not be healthy as well?

The approach that a lot of people take with health is more is better. As it relates to exercise, that is not the case [233]. I often hear clients say, "I guess I just need to exercise more". It is like a reflex. If they had been working out 45 minutes a day, they will just increase to 90 minutes a day. Clearly, exercise in the sedentary is beneficial [234]. But exercise does have a plateau in benefit: a point at which exercise loses its benefits and crosses the line to detriment. And this is where the negative health benefits are found in these extreme levels of training.

Two studies prove this point. The first was published in Lancet in 2012. The authors of this study found a plateau of reduced mortality with exercise [235]. The plateau point occurred at 50 minutes

233  O'Keefe JH, Patil HR, Lavie CJ, Magalski A, Vogel RA, McCullough PA. Potential adverse cardiovascular effects from excessive endurance exercise. Mayo Clinic Proceedings. June 2012;87(6):587-595.

234  Wen CP et al. Minimum amount of physical activity for reduced mortality and extended life expectancy: a prospective cohort study. Lancet. 2011;378(9798):1244-1253.

235  O'Keefe JH, Patil HR, Lavie CJ. Exercise and life expectancy. Lancet. 2012;379(9818):799.

of strenuous exercise. Beyond 50 minutes, the health benefits of exercise started to plateau and become stagnant. See below graph.

The second study was also published in 2012. This study looked at 52,656 adults and all-cause mortality. What they found was that health benefits occurred in those running up to 19.9 miles/week at speeds of 6-7 miles/hour, 2 to 5 times weekly [236]. Beyond that point, no further reduction in mortality was found. Again, there is a plateau of benefits with exercise. More is not better. It is beyond this "plateau" that damage ensues.

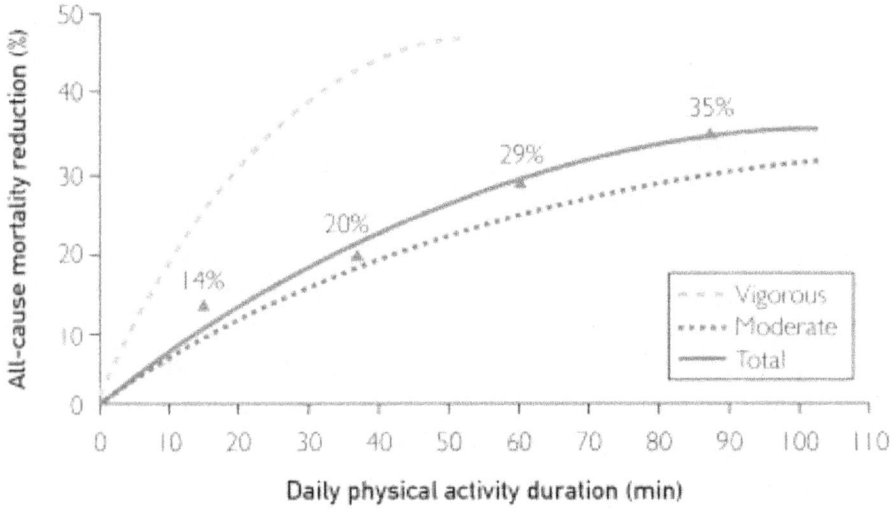

*(Figure 1 plateau of benefits from all-cause mortality with exercise )*[22]

The proposed mechanism of harm in extreme training is heart muscle damage, fibrosis of the heart, and resultant cardiac dysfunction. A very well documented animal study replicated this. The rats were exposed to strenuous exercise for 60 minutes daily for 4 months. What the authors of the study found, was: hypertrophy of the left ventricle and the right ventricle, diastolic dysfunction,

---

236   Lee J, Patte R, Lavie CH, Blair SN. Running and all-cause mortality risk: is more better? Med Sci Sports Exerc. 2012;44(6):990-994.

dilation of the left and right atrium, and fibrosis of the heart atria and ventricles [237]. Similar findings of enlarged heart, enlarged heart ventricles, and increased atrial size have been found in high intensity exercise in humans as well [238] [239].

When you look at marathon runners, the risk of sudden cardiac death is rare at 1:100,000 [240]. The rate is slightly higher in triathletes at 1.5:100,000 [241]. Is there evidence of cardiac damage? Is their evidence of damage to the heart in marathon runners, triathletes, and the like? The answer is yes. Several biomarkers of cardiac damage to include cardiac troponin, creatine kinase MB, and BNP have been shown to increase 50% in runners following a marathon [24] [28] [29] [242]. And some of this damage results in cardiac muscular changes, previously stated scarring and fibrosis, that appear to be irreversible [243]. Some of these biomarker elevations and muscle remodeling is normal in regular exercise. But, in these extreme forms of exercise, these biomarker elevations and muscle remodeling also becomes extreme level and the effects are lasting and irreversible.

James H. O'keefe, MD is one of the leading experts in the world on the negative cardiovascular effects of extreme exercise. He is a former extreme athlete himself, but has since changed due to the growing body of evidence on the negative effects of this extreme

237  Michaelides Ap et al. Exercise duration as a determinant of vascular function and antioxidant balance in patients with coronary artery disease. Heart. 2011;97(10):832-837.

238  Pelliccia A, Culasso F, Di Paolo FM, Maron BJ. Physiologic left ventricular cavity dilation in elite athletes. Ann Intern Med. 1999;130(1):23-31.

239  Pelliccia et al. Prevalence and clinical significance of left atrial remodeling in competitive athletes. J Am Coll Cardiol. 2005;46(4):690-696.

240  Redelmeier DA, Greenwald JA. Competing risks of mortality with marathons: retrospective analysis. BMJ. 2007;335(7633):1275-1277.

241  Harris KM et al. Sudden death during the Triathlon. JAMA. 2010;303(13):1255-1257.

242  Kim JH et al. Cardiac arrest during long-distance running races. N Engl J Med. 2012;366(2):130-140.

243  La Gerche A et al. Exercise-induced right ventricular dysfunction and structural remodeling in endurance athletes. Eur Heart. 2012;33(8):995-1006.

training. Dr. O'Keefe published a great review article describing the cardiovascular damage from excessive exercise can be found in the 2012 Mayo Clinic Proceedings [21]. In fact, Dr O'keefe warns men 40 to avoid triathlons all together.

So, exercise and athletics don't always translate to "healthy". I often tell our clients that with weight loss, I want the focus to be different. I don't want the client to lose weight to be healthy: I want the client to be healthy to lose weight. Many focus on losing weight, and they do. But, they don't achieve the weight loss through health, and of course rebound with weight gain. The same applies to exercise. I want exercise to contribute to a client's health, not become a detriment to health.

Client's that come in to our office to lose weight often focus on exercise. I usually throw them a curve ball by telling them that I want to wait on exercise. First we need to improve their biochemistry so that they will see the full benefit of their exercise. Many who come to our office could not handle the stressors of exercise, even a simple exercise regimen would overtax their physiology. Many come in a catabolic state. Meaning: their body is in active break down mode. There is no healing and regeneration ongoing. Only breakdown and destruction exists. If their body is already in an active break down mode, why would I want to add to that with exercise. In that instance, we change their physiology to one of an anabolic state (building mode) from the catabolic state and then add in exercise. That way, they will benefit from exercise and eliminate the potential negative side effects.

The perfect example is a client JS. He came in with complaints of fatigue and inability to lose weight. He had tried everything from prescription diet pills to the HCG diet and everything else in between. He found no consistent weight loss in his attempts. In fact, he had gained weight over the 2 year interval of weight loss attempts. His metabolic test results revealed, in addition to significant hormone abnormalities, muscle breakdown, mitochondrial dysfunction, oxidative stress, and poor nutritional balance. Add that to his 13% muscle content. That is right–13%. This client was in absolutely no physiological place to handle or see the benefits of exercise. In fact, if he did start a significant exercise regimen, he would likely accelerate his muscle breakdown and further compromise his ability to burn fat.

The body's ability to burn fat is concentrated within mitochondria. Mitochondria are found throughout most cells of the body, but particularly muscle. Mitochondria are the power houses of the cell. Mitochondria's primary role is in energy production. Low muscle content equals low mitochondrial content. JS had low capacity to burn fat due to his low muscle mass and thus low mitochondrial content. JS needed to improve mitochondrial and muscle content first. Increasing muscle and mitochondrial content in JS would improve his capacity to burn calories. Starting off with heavy cardio work outs would not help JS build more muscle and mitochondria. Cardio at this stage, will only lead to further muscle breakdown, further muscle loss, continued loss/compromise of mitochondrial function, and continued weight gain. This example is not uncommon with either men or women.

Let's look at another example. JF was soccer coach and an avid soccer player. In his off days, JF competed in an amateur soccer league. He was very fit and very active. No one would question JF's health. He was not overweight by any stretch yet he struggled with energy. He knew that he could perform better and knew he could just feel better. How JF felt did not agree with how he was told how he should feel. Evaluation revealed hormone imbalances–low Testosterone and increased Estrogen production. Additionally, mitochondrial dysfunction was found. Both, will hamper recovery from training. As a result he was in a pro-inflammatory state and a mild catabolic state. We instituted mitochondrial support and aromatase inhibition (inhibits Testosterone to Estrogen production). Changed him from a pro-inflammatory state to a anti-inflammatory state and improved mitochondrial function, reversing the catabolic state into an anabolic state, reversing the breakdown mode to building mode. The result was weight loss and resolution of his energy problems. Now he is playing soccer with men, in some cases, half his age.

All this negativity on exercise, one would think that I am against exercise. The opposite is true. I exercise 4-5 days weekly. I love exercise. However, I am a huge proponent for customized exercise at the right time in the right amount. Just as a one-size-fits-all approach doesn't work for hormones, it doesn't work for exercise either.

There are many benefits of exercise. The benefits from exercise [244], far outweigh the risks for most.

- Exercise improves muscle performance and oxygen utilization by tissue. This is even found in those with cardiovascular disease [245] [246] [247]. The cardiovascular system becomes more efficient.
- Exercise improves the anaerobic threshold [248]. This results in improved performance.

---

244 Fletcher GF et al. Statement on Exercise: Benefits and Recommendations for Physical Activity Programs for all Americans. Circulation. 1996;94:857-862.

245 Kobashigawa JA, Leaf DA, Gleeson MP et al. Benefit of cardiac rehabiltation in heart transplant patients: a randomized trial. J Heart Lung Transplant. 1994;90:S77.

246 Kavanagh T, Yacoub MH, Mertens DJ, Kennedy J, Campbell RB, Sawyer P. Cardiorespiratory responses to exercise training after orthotopic cardiac transplantation. Circulation. 1988;77:162-171.

247 Hambrecht R et al. Physical training in patients with stable chronic heart failure: effects on cardiorespiratory fitness and ultrastructural abnormalities of leg muscles. J Am Coll Cardiol. 1995;25:1239-1249.

248 Sullivan MJ, Higginbotham MB, Cobb FR. Exercise training in patients with chronic heart failure delays ventilatory anaeorbic threshold and improves

- Exercise improves the cardiovascular oxygen utilization. The cardiovascular system becomes a more efficient user of oxygen [249] and the rate of decline in oxygen utilization is slowed [250].
- Exercise improves high density lipoproteins (HDL) [251]. HDL is the often claimed "good cholesterol". There is really no such thing, but according to the Framingham study [252], an increased total Cholesterol to HDL ratio is associated with an increase in cardiovascular disease (CVD). Increase the HDL content of that equation and one will lower that ratio and lower the risk of CVD.
- Exercise improves fat distribution in men of all ages [253] and can. result in a significant decline in weight, percent body fat, and fat mass.
- Exercise reduces cardiovascular disease risk [254].
- Exercise reduces mortality risk in those individuals with cardiovascular disease [255] [256].

submaximal exercise performance. Circulation. 1989;79:324-329.

249 Trap-Jensen J, Clausen JP. Effect of training on the relation of heart rate and blood pressure to the onset of painin effort angina pectoris. In: Larsen OA, Malmborg RO, eds. Coraonary Heart Disease and Physical Fitness: Symposium on Physical Fitness and Coronary Heart Disease. Baltimore, Md: University Park Press; 1971:111-114.

250 Jackson AS, Beard EF, Wier LT, Ross RM, Stutevill JE, Blair SN. Changes in aerobic power of men, ages 25-70 yr. Med Sci Sports Exerc. 1995;27:113-120.

251 Tran ZV, Weltman A. Differential effects of exercise on serum lipid and lipoprotein levels seen with changes in body weight: a meta-analysis. JAMA. 1985;254:919-924.

252 Linn S, Fulwood R, Carroll M, Brook JG, Johnson C, Kalsbeek WD, Rifkind BM. Serum total cholesterol: HDL cholesterol ratios in US white and black adults by selected demographic and socioeconomic variables (HANES II). Am J Public health. Aug 1991;81(8):1038-43.

253 Schwartz RS et al. The effect of intensive endurance exercise training on body fat distribution in young and older men. Metabolism. 1991;40:545-551.

254 Donahue RP, Abbott RD, Bloom E, Reed DM, Yao K. Central obesity and coronary heart disease in men. Lancet. 1987;1:821-824.

255 O'Connor GT et al. An overview of randomized trials of rehabilitation with exercise after myocardial infarction. Circulation. 1989;80:234-244.

256 Oldridge NB, Guyatt GH. Fischer ME, Rimm AA. Cardiac rehabilitation after myocardial infarction: combined experience of randomized clinical trials. JAMA. 1988;260:945-950.

- Exercise improves insulin sensitivity [257] [258].
- Exercise reduces fibrinogen levels in men [259].
- Exercise has been shown to reduce the incidence of colon cancer [260] and breast [261] cancer by 30-40%.
- Exercise was found to increase the life expectancy by 7 years[262] and reduce disability [263].
- Exercise improves glucose utilization and body composition through improved basal metabolism [264] [265].
- Exercise improves muscular performance and builds bones [266].
- Exercise improves quality of life [267] [268]. I don't know what is more important than that.

257 King DS et al. Effects of exercise and lack of exercise on insulin sensitivity and responsiveness. J Appl Physiol. 1988;64:1942-1946.

258 Rosenthal M, Haskell WL, Solomon R, Widstrom A, Reaven GM. Demonstration of a relationship between level of physical training and insulin-stimulated glucose utilization normal humans. Diabetes. 1983;32:408-411.

259 Stratton JR et al. Effects of physical conditioning on fibrinolytic variables and fibrinogen in young and old healthy adults. Circulation. 1991;83:1692-1697.

260 Lee IM. Physical activity, fitness, and cancer. In: Bouchard C, Shephard RN, Stephens T, eds. Physical Activity, Fitness, and Health: International Proceedings and Consensus Statement. Champaign, Ill: Human Kinetics Publishers; 1994:814-831.

261 Lee l-Min. Physical activity and cancer prevention-data from epidemiologic studies. Medicine and Science in sports and exercise. 2003;35(11):1823-1827.

262 Sarna S, Sahi T, Koskenvuo M, Kaprio J. Increased life expectancy of world class male athletes. Med Sci Sports Exerc. 1993;25:237-44.

263 Chakravarty EF et al. Reduced disability and mortality among aging runners. JAMA Internal Medicine. 2008;168(15):1638-1646.

264 Kohrt WM, Holloszy JO. Loss of skeletal muscle mass with aging: effect on glucose tolerance. J Geronto A Biol Scie Med Sci. 1995;50:68-72.

265 Evans WJ. Effects of exercise on body composition and functional capacity of the elderly. J Gerontol A Biol Scie Med Sci. 1995;50:147-150.

266 ACSM position stand on osteoporosis and exercise: American College of Sports Medicine. Med Sci Sports Exerc. 1995;27:1-7.

267 Stewart KJ, Mason M, Keleman MH. Three-year participation in circuit weight training improves muscular strength and self-efficacy in cardiac patients. J Cardiopulmonary Rehabil. 1998;8:292-296.

268 Sparling PB, Cantwell JD, Dolan CM, Niderman RK. Strength training in a cardiac rehabilitation program: a six-month follow-up. Arch Phys Med Rehabil. 1990;71:148-152.

- Regular exercise is associated with being better "adjusted" [269].
- Exercise improves cognitive functioning [270].
- Exercise improves the physiologic response to stressors [271] [272].
- Exercise is associated with a reduction in anxiety and depression symptoms [273].
- Exercise doesn't just help with depressive symptoms, exercise helps to reduce the incidence of depression in healthy [274] and non-healthy [275] [276] individuals.
- Exercise improves self image through improved self-confidence and improved self-esteem [277].

Clearly, in moderation, exercise has tremendous benefits. What does the scientific evidence say about what is the best form of exercise? Not, what is your physician's opinion on the best form of exercise. Not what is everybody doing, or what does your personal trainer say. But, what does the scientific data say on what exercise provides the best benefit?

---

269 Eysenck HJ, Nias DKB, Cox DN. Sport and personality. Adv Behav Res Ther. 1982;4:1-56.

270 Spirduso WW. Physical fitness, aging, and psychomotor speed: a review. J Gerontol. 1980;35:850-865.

271 Crews DJ, Landers DM. A meta-analytic review of aerobic fitness and reactivity to psychosocial stressor. Med Sci Sports Exerc. 1987;19:S114-S120.

272 Blumenthal et al. Aerobic exercise reduces levels of cardiovascular and sympathoadrenal responses to mental stress in subjects without prior evidence of myocardial ischemia. Am J Cardiol. 1990;65:93-98.

273 Lobstein DD, Mosbacher BJ, Ismail AH. Depressino as a powerful discriminator between physicaly active and sedentary middle-aged men. J Psychosom Res. 1983;27:69-76.

274 Blumenthal JA et al. Cardiovascular and behavioral effects of aeorbic exercise training in healthy older men and women. J Gerontol. 1989;44:M147-M157.

275 Kavanagh T, Shephard RJ, Tuck JA, Qureshi S. Depression following myocardial infarction: the effects of distance running. Ann NY Acad Sci. 1977;301:1029-1038.

276 Martinsen EW, Medhus A, Sandvik L. Effects of aeorbic exercise on depression: a controlled study. Br Med J (Clin Res Ed). 1985;291:109.

277 Folkins CH, Sime WE. Physical fitness training and mental health. Am J Psychol. 1981;36:373-389.

To prove my point here, there was a recent public seminar in our home town on health. They had 2 physicians speak on health. Neither physician was the "appearance of health" and in fact one of the physicians said he needed to take his own advice and start exercising. Where is the credibility in that? They were speaking on health, yet neither physician followed what they, themselves were preaching.

Again, what does the science say. Not, what does public opinion say.

Of course exercise is beneficial. However, exercise needs to match the individual's metabolic needs. When time is of the essence and weight-loss is the goal, according to a recent study, cardio is the best, with a mix of cardio/resistance the second best, and resistance training only as the 3rd best [278]. So, in those individuals doing nothing, doing anything, but particularly cardio exercise is a great place to start. If one is already performing regular cardio exercise, then add in resistance training 1-2 times weekly at 30 minutes each.

Don't think you need to start training for a marathon or 1/2 marathon. Simple cardio will work. This should be under the guidance of a medical provider or personal trainer to avoid injury. Start simple and increase gradually. Walking, jogging, ellipticals, cross country skiing and the like are great forms of cardio exercise. Another great program for those doing nothing is the program "Couch to 5-K". This provides a structured, gentle approach to move from a sedentary lifestyle to an active lifestyle.

This brings me to the next point. You must have a goal. You must set short-term and long-term goals. Without goals, you will have

278  Willis LH et al. Effects of aerobic and/or resistance training on body mass and fat mass in overweight or obese adults. Journal of Applied Physiology. Dec 15 2012;113(12):1831-1837.

no focus. Without focus, you will achieve nothing. It has been shown that 50% of those that start exercise programs, will continue them for more than 6 months [279]. Guys, I hate to say this, but my experience are that we guys comply more with this statistic than do the ladies.

Don't think you will reach your goal of a 5k in 3 months. Be realistic. Be persistent and stay focused on your goals. The short-term goals will allow you to see the progress. Sometimes the mountain to overcome seems so great that the mere presence of the mountain provides reason to quit. But, short steps make the insurmountable achievable. It took me about 4 years to achieve my almost 100 lb weight loss. But I have kept it off for 10+ years now. Health doesn't just happen. Being fit doesn't just happen. It requires work, effort, and goals. It requires a life style change. One cannot reverse a lifetime of poor health in just a fraction of the time it took to get to the state of poor health.

Back to the question at hand. What form of exercise is best? There will be varying of opinion between experts. But when time is short and results are at a premium (which is the case for most of us), then high-intensity interval training (HIT) is the best. High-intensity interval training is a mix of short, intense exercise followed by less intense recovery phase. An example would be 30 seconds of sprinting followed by 60 seconds of walking. Then repeat this cycle multiple times. But don't think that you have to start off with sprints. Start with fast walking, but follow the mix of intervals. Even the Couch to 5k starts with an interval of 60 seconds of jogging followed by 90 seconds of walking. Just get started with the jogging and work your way up to the sprints.

---

279  Dishman RK. Compliance/adherence in health related exercise. Health Psychol. 1982;1237-267.

Below is an example we hand out to our clients. But if this seems too much, that is ok. Cut the reps and time intervals in half, or more. The point, is get started!:

Studies reveal that HIT provides similar benefits to endurance training in a shorter amount of time [280]. High-intensity interval training has even shown to be beneficial in older adults [281]. How? High-intensity interval training has been shown to increase mitochondrial capacity and performance [282]. Remember, mitochondria are the "power house" of the cell. The capacity to make energy is found in the mitochondria in the cell. So, it stands to reason that if you increase the capacity to make energy, you increase the capacity to burn fat. In fact, a 2 week session of 7 intervals of HIT in women, was found to increase the muscular mitochondrial capacity to burn fat through fatty acid oxidation [283]. The previously referenced study from the Journal of Physiology, found the same to be true for men. They found that HIT exercise increased muscular mitochondrial capacity, improved exercise performance, improved insulin sensitivity, and improved markers (Sirt1 and PGC-1alpha) that point to increased mitochondrial production by 56% [70]. When it comes to time commitment and physiologic results, it is hard pressed to beat that of high-intensity interval training.

Again, if the above example is too much. That is ok. Just cut the reps and time intervals in half. The point, is get started!

280   Gibala MJ, Little JP, MacDonald MJ, Hawley JA. Physiological adaptations to low-volume, high-intensity interval training in health and disease. The Journal of Physiology. Mar 1, 2012;590:1077-1084.

281   Whitehurst M. High-intensity interval training: An alternative for older adults. American Journal of Lifestyle Medicine. Sept/Oct 2012;6(5):382-386.

282   Little JP et al. A practical model of low-volume high-intensity interval training induces mitochondrial biogeneisis in human skeletal muscle: potential mechanism. The Journal of Physiology. Mar 15 2010;588:1011-1022.

283   Talanian JL et al. Two weeks of high-intensity aerobic interval training increases the capacity for fat oxidation during exercise in women. Journal of Applied Physiology. April 2007;102(4):1439-1447.

Finally, what if I told you that genetics plays a role in the benefits of exercise? There is genetic testing available that allows your provider to prescribe exercise to match your genetics makeup to maximize your physiologic benefits. These genetic tests allow us to customize exercise for maximum metabolic effect. For example, some individuals receive much more benefit from cardio training. Where as others need a heavy dose of resistance training. A genetic evaluation by your provider can determine which will work best for you.

Think of that, a prescription of metabolic efficiency! Wild, but these are the times we live in. We are a product of our genetics and our environment. When the two work together we get great results. When they don't, well...Just look around you. Today we have the capacity to test both the genetic predisposition and the current physiological function to prescribe the best, customized program for each individual. No longer do we have to guess and maybe get it right. We can prescribe a plan for each client from the beginning and remove every obstacle except for the individual.

In conclusion, exercise is great in the right amounts and for the right metabolic reasons. As it relates to testosterone, proper exercise aids the metabolic benefit of testosterone. Lack of exercise is a contributor to a slowed metabolism and thus weight gain. With weight gain comes increased estrogen production, which decreases testosterone production. However, excessive exercise as in OTS can contribute to low testosterone. So, with any treatment strategy, balance is the key. The key question is where are you?

# CHAPTER 8

# HORMONES

"Brevity is the soul of wit"–Shakespeare

It only takes a pill. It just needs to be cut out. It is all about Testosterone... Simple. When it comes to health care, simple is the modus operendi. Simple would be nice. Simple, would be... well, simple. But, the body does not work on simple. Simple is men are nothing but testosterone fueled erections and when we hit empty on the ole testosterone gauge, we just stop off at the local testosterone dispenser and we are good to go–"filler up!" But, the body is an incredibly dynamic biological organism. And though they may seem simple enough, they are really a complex biochemical machine maintaining an intricate, delicate, balance.

The medical establishment would have you think your body is linear. That Hypertension is itself a disease of the arteries. That Diabetes is a disease of sugar and the pancreas. That obesity is merely a product of too many calories in and not enough calories out (I actually had a physician on the Louisiana state board tell me that–the lack of knowledge was frightening). That is linear thinking and only partially true. But, I want you to step outside the box and look at you body's biochemistry through a different light. To focus on solutions in disease, not band-aids. To focus on pathways to health restoration, not disease management. If one only seeks to manage disease, how can one ever restore health?

Hormones are a good example of this linear thinking. Women are just a sponge of Estrogen and men are just a body full of Testosterone. You may laugh, but look at the therapies offered today. Look at the commercials these days. Middle aged men with good Testosterone dancing with their shadows. All his strength, energy, and vigor restored. And of course, good sexual function results in long golf drives admired by all your friends. Or the latest, men walking around looking "1.62%" larger than life with a "10$ prescription" (as if you health is only worth 10$). The advertisement may bring a chuckle, but cheap, simple solutions are not funny, they are dangerous.

Don't get me wrong. Low Testosterone is a very common problem in men today. But it is also a very complex problem. Yes Virginia, men are complex. It is not just about low testosterone, but it is more about what causes low T that makes it complex. The causes of low T are diverse: and in that diversity, we find the expanded impact of low T.

Today's relativism has blurred the lines between black and white, between truth and fiction. It doesn't really matter if people still think that the earth is flat (believe it or not, there is a world is flat society), the earth is in fact round. Have you seen a NASA photo of earth lately? Or more relevant to this discussion, have you seen the biochemical pathways?

All that to say that "simple" would be nice. But our body is quite complex. We shouldn't be surprised, because we are "beautifully and wonderfully made".

Brevity is great when your focus is wit, but rarely equates to brevity in the complex world of biochemistry.

Hormones are such an example of the complex. When I discuss hormones and results of hormone testing with people, I highlight 5 points on hormones:

- hormone levels
- hormone balance
- hormone metabolism
- hormone receptors
- outside influences

It takes all these to get symptom resolution and good physiologic function. Again, your Testosterone doesn't exist in a bottle. Rather, Testosterone is just one important piece (and a very important piece at that) of a puzzle influenced and effected by many variables. But, it takes all pieces of the puzzle to give you a clear finished product.

So what is Testosterone? Testosterone is the predominate hormone in men. From the beginning, Testosterone is the key to male development. It is what makes a man a man. It is what gave us Tim the tool man Taylor from the 1990's sitcom, Home Improvement.

Then what is low T? Quite simply, it is low Testosterone. Low T is fatigue, low T is reduced libido, low T is ED, low T is weight gain, and Low T is loss of confidence and motivation. I think you get the picture. Low T is all around us, but it presents itself in many different forms. Low T is in many ways the middle-aged man suffering the dreaded "mid-life crisis". Think about it. What is happening to women about the same time? Men can be just as hormonal as women; we just don't like to admit it. Men hormonal? Yup. We just express it differently.

Low Testosterone is a lot more common than you think. The estimates are that 5 to 10% of men suffer from low T [284] [285] [286]. The problem with these studies is that the authors subscribe to the concept that men are just testosterone fueled erections. These large studies only considered the men with "loss of morning erections, low sexual desire, and erectile dysfunction" as symptomatic of low T [287]. Translated: only men with sexual dysfunction were included in their study on low T. However, when you consider the "non-sexual" symptoms, the levels approach an estimated 40 million, rather than 4.7 million. Only a fraction of these 40 million men are symptomatic. Which means that most of the men that are walking around with low T, don't even know it.

Don't you just love surprises? Not at age 30 you don't. Not only is low T a silent problem, but also it is a growing problem. More and more men at younger and younger ages are discovering they have low T. I've seen men in their mid-20's with low Testosterone. However, most men I see are in their 40's and beyond.

If only the cause of low T was low Testosterone production. Life would be simple, life would be easy, and life would be good. But look at our bodies–we are complex creations. In fact, in most cases, low T is the symptom. It is the effect and not the cause.

Women are told the cure to their hormone symptoms is removal of their uterus and ovaries and then their fountain of youth is estrogen replacement–right. That is what I was told to say and that is

---

284  Araujo AB et al. Prevalence and Incidence of androgen deficiency in middle-aged and older men: estimates fromt eh Massachusetts Male Aging Study. Journal of Clinical Endocrinology and Metabolism. Dec 2004;89(12):5920-5926.

285  Araujo AB et al. Prevalence of symptomatic androgen deficiency in men. Journal of Clinical Endocrinology and Metabolism. Nov 2007;92(11):4241-4247.

286  Wu FC et al. Identification of Late-Onset Hypogonadism in Middle-Aged and Elderly Men. New England Journal of Medicine. June 16 2010.

287  Araujo AB, Wittert GA. Endocrinology of the Aging Mle. Best Pract Res Clin Endocrinol Metab. April 2011;25(2):303-319.

what I used to say. So, if we follow the same logic in men, then men's cure to low T should be removal of a man's…. I can't bring myself to say it. Would any man gladly agree or even entertain that as a viable option?!

The point is, the causes of hormone imbalances in women and the causes of low T in men are dynamic. Sure, low T is the direct cause of decreased production of testosterone from the male gonads. But why? What is the cause?

Remember the old saying, "you are what you eat". That couldn't be more appropriate to this subject. Today, we eat so many items that suppress the body's natural testosterone production. Just look at the amount of sugar that we eat today. Americans eat up to 200 lbs of refined sugar and 90 lbs of fats annually. This would equate to 63 dozen donuts, 60 lbs of cakes and cookies, 23 gallons of ice cream, 22 lbs of candy, and 15 lbs of chips, popcorn, and pretzels annually. If that won't make you sick, I don't know what will. The point is, this leads to excess weight. This excess weight, especially around the mid section, becomes a major Estrogen pro-ducing factory for men. It has been estimated that 80% of estrogen production in men comes from abdominal fat [288].

Not only, does the associated weight gain help produce more Estrogen, but the enzyme (aromatase) that converts testosterone to Estrogen increases as we age as well. All this said, we men become a little to in touch with our feminine side. We become estrogen dominant. And what is important about excess estrogen? The excess estrogen leads to decrease testosterone production through inhibition of the hypothalamus and pituitary stimulation of tes-tosterone production from the testes. This is one of the primary causes of low T.

---

288  Vermeulen A, Kaufman JM, Goemaere S, van Pottelberg I. Estradiol in elderly men. Aging Male. Jun 2002;5(2):98-102.

# HIGH-INTENSITY INTERVAL TRAINING

## First 2 weeks

- sprint as fast as you can for 30 seconds
- followed by interval walk at normal pace for 60 secs
- perform 5 reps 3 times weekly

## Week 2 - 4

- sprint as fast as you can for 45 seconds
- followed by interval walk at normal pace for 60 seconds
- perform 5 reps 3 x weekly

## Week 4 - 6

- sprint as fast as you can for 60 seconds
- followed by interval walk at normal pace for 60 seconds
- perform 5 reps 3 x weekly

## Week 6 - 8

- sprint as fast as you can for 60 seconds
- followed by interval walk at normal pace for 60 seconds
- perform 10 reps 3 x weekly

The growing obesity epidemic is a major contributor to the low T problem today. According to the CDC, 35.7% of Americans today are obese, with another 33% overweight. Add those up and you get a whopping 2/3 of Americans are obese or overweight. Remember: obesity equal excess estrogen production which results in low T.

The Environment is another contributor to low T. The environment is full of hormone-like chemicals called xenoestrogens. Xenoestrogens are environmental estrogens that literally mean foreign Estrogens. Xenoestrogens can range from pesticides/insecticides to plastics to hormone-laden meat and dairy products. They may be foreign to the body, but the body views them as Estrogens nonetheless. And we all know what that means: estrogen dominance and low Testosterone.

Hormones can be another source of low T. That's right. Even giving Testosterone to some men can be a problem. I can recall a 27-year man that was given Testosterone for a suspected low T problem. The Testosterone replacement made him feel worse. Why? He was already Estrogen dominant (that was the cause of his low T). His biochemistry was already making large volumes of Estrogen from his endogenous Testosterone production. His high Testosterone to Estrogen production actually was the inhibiting Testosterone production at the level of the hypothalamus and pituitary. The Testosterone that he was given was just like throwing gasoline on the fire. His suspected cure, Testosterone, turned out to be fuel for the source of his problem—excess estrogen. This reminds me of many of the "low T" commercials. Most of the men in these commercials, as are most men today, are overweight. So, Testosterone therapy in these men is just throwing fuel on the fire.

So, how does one properly evaluate hormones?

There is a lot of debate these days about the different methods to evaluate hormones: blood, saliva, and urine (oh my...). You would think that this debate would center around the science of the different methods of testing. Sadly, that couldn't be further from the truth.

Many highly respected researchers and clinicians have written on the advantages and disadvantages of the different test mediums [289]. It is about perspective.

A good friend of mine uses the analogy of FedEx trucks to explain this difference in perspective. FedEx trucks are everywhere during the month of December. It wouldn't be unusual for a lot of trucks to pass your house during that month. But, if the FedEx trucks don't stop at your house it doesn't really matter how many trucks have driven by your house or how many packages each truck contained–none stopped for delivery. It only takes one truck to stop and the Christmas tree is full. I'll take it one step further. The day after Christmas the boxes and wrapping paper start to pile up at the road-side for pickup. You might comment as you drive by your neighbors house, "looks like the Jones' had a good Christmas" based on the aftermath. You can even make out what the gifts were based on the left over debris curbside.

The point is that the FedEx trucks are the hormones in transport in the blood. It doesn't matter how many hormones are transported through the blood (FedEx trucks), these are inactive. These packages (hormones) are locked up in the truck unavailable for you to enjoy.

The truck stopping at the house delivering the presents inside your home is hormones in the saliva. The package is delivered inside the cell (the house) to be enjoyed. What matters is how many hormones are dropped off for action inside the cell. One

---

289  Zava D. Saliva Hormone Testing. Townsend Letter. Jan 2004.

truck can drop off 100 packages or 100 trucks can drive by dropping off no packages.

Finally, the driveway debris post-Christmas represent the hormones in the urine. The body eliminates the hormones through the urine as breakdown metabolites through the process of hormone metabolism.

Remember, it is all about perspective.

Now, that you understand the perspective of the different tests. What does the science say about blood, saliva, and urine?

There has been a battle brewing in medicine over this. Equally, there has been a growing body of evidence over the past 30-40 years. Unfortunately, a lot of the medical governing bodies have locked themselves in closets and have refused to look at the scientific data available and objectively debate the science.

Just recently, it was published that 42-51% of Americans will be obese by 2030 [290] (up from 15% in 1970). And according to the United Health Foundations rankings, Louisiana and Mississippi rank 49 and 50 respectively. Louisiana was 47 just 2 years earlier. According to 2012 data, Louisiana just moved back to the 50th position to beat out Mississippi and claim the distinction of the fattest state in the union.

I guess they take the philosophy: "if it ain't broke, don't fix it". In the medical vernacular, that is called "standard practice". The definition of standard practice is what the majority are doing. But, according to statistics, "standard practice" is only increasing the standard level of disease and poor health. Sorry, it is broke and it desperately needs fixing. And current, documented

---

290  Finkelstein EA et al. Obesity and severe obesity forecasts through 2030. Am J Prev Med. 2012.

scientific research must be the source of that fix. So let's look at the research.

## Blood Testing

Hormone testing through the blood has been the only game in town for a long time. This form of testing has been used to develop the current reference norms for the diagnosis and managements of many diseases today. And, this method is effective in the disease model of medicine when physiology breaks down. However, the wellness model of medicine searches for dysfunction, not just absolute disease. This is where traditional blood testing breaks down. By identifying physiologic dysfunction, the wellness model hopes to prevent disease.

Make no mistake, this is nothing short of true preventative medicine. Certainly we must and will continue to treat disease. And disease is best treated if detected early. But better still is to prevent disease before it begins through wellness. Identifying physiologic dysfunction is where blood hormone testing fails.

The problem with blood hormone testing is three fold. First, is the whole needle thing. Hey, if you can evaluate levels without puncturing the skin, it is a good idea. Second, blood testing evaluates the total levels and then calculates the "free", active hormone levels via a formula with several variables. Most of the hormone in the blood is protein bound (estimated at 95-99% [291]) and inactive. As a physician, this does me very little good to evaluate transported, inactive hormones then calculate the active hormones. Why not just cut to the chase and check the active hormones? Most important, there is a better way. Saliva testing is proving to be superior to blood testing for hormones (see below).

---

291   Azad RM. Abnormal serum thyroid hormones concentration with healthy functional gland: a review on the metabolic role of thyroid hormones transporter proteins. Pak J Biol Sci. Mar 1 2011;14(5):313-26.

## Urine Testing

The use of urine to evaluate cortisol has been present for awhile. And this is a valid method to test cortisol. The problem is, most people don't want to have to carry a jug around to collect urine for 24 hours. Currently, the interesting research on urinary testing of hormones is in the metabolites via dried urine.

Cortisol metabolism has been shown to play a role in chronic fatigue syndrome (CFS) and in obesity. Low cortisol, especially low morning cortisol [292], has been associated with CFS. The majority of studies reveal low adrenal cortisol output as a primary physiologic finding. However, new studies suggest hyper-metabolism may play a role in those with CFS. So, in those with low cortisol as in chronic fatigue, the problem with the low cortisol may be hyper-metabolism [293] and the excessive removal of cortisol. This suggests high adrenal output with equally high metabolism of cortisol. Many would call low cortisol adrenal fatigue or hypoadrenia, but with high stress, the body increases the metabolism of cortisol and this can be found through evaluation of urinary metabolites. This can only be assessed by evaluation of cortisol and cortisol metabolites. Currently, urine is the only medium to be able to evaluate both simultaneously.

In the CFS example, therapy to increase cortisol would actually be the wrong approach. The body is actually trying to protect against high cortisol by increasing metabolism and elimination of excess cortisol. Increasing cortisol production is going against the body. The appropriate therapy would be to reduce stress. An additional benefit of urinary metabolites is evaluation of cortisol metabolism

---

292   Cleare AJ, Miell J, Heap E, Sookdeo S, Young L, Malhi GS, O'Keane V. Hypothalamo-Pituitary-Adrenal Axis Dysfunction in Chronic Fatigue Syndrome and the Effects of Low-Dose Hydorcortisone therapy. JCEM. Aug 1 2001;86(8):3545-3554.

293   Jeries WK et al. Urinary Cortisol and Cortisol metabolite excretion in chronic fatigue syndrome. Psychosomatic Medicine. July 1 2006;68(4):578-582.

in fat [294]. This process plays a role in the development of insulin resistance, metabolic syndrome, and obesity.

Estrogen metabolite testing is not new. The pathways of estrogen metabolism are via the 2-OH-estrone, 16-alpha-OH-estrone, and 4-OH estrone pathways. Some research has suggested that the ratio of 2-OH-estrone:16-alpha-OH-estrone [295] is predictive of breast cancer risk. A recent review of 9 studies [296] involving 2,915 people did not support this hypothesis. So, the jury is still out on the benefit of that ratio. What is well supported throughout the literature is the dangers present in the 4-OH-estrone pathway [297]. This pathway is associated with an increased breast, and prostate [298] cancer risk.

Let's give progesterone equal time. Many of you may be familiar with the oral progesterone metabolite, allo-alpha-pregnanolone. Well, you may not be, but this metabolite is the reason that oral progesterone helps you sleep. How you take progesterone effects the metabolism of progesterone.

In contrast, transdermal progesterone provides very little urinary metabolites (better evaluated in saliva) [299] compared to oral pro-

---

294  Roberge C et al. Adrenocortical dysregulation as a major player in insulin resistance and onset of obesity. AJP-Endo. Dec 2007;293(6):E1465-E1478.

295  Im A et al. Urinary estrogen metabolites in women at high risk for breast cancer. Carcinogenesis. 2009;30(9):1532-1535.

296  Obi N, Vrieling A, Heinz J, Chang-Claude J. Estrogen metabolite ratio: Is the 2-hydroestone to 16-alpha-hydroxyestrone ratio predictive for breast cancer? Int J Women's Health. 2011;3:37-51.

297  Gaikwad NW et al. Urine biomarkers of risk in the molecular etiology of Breast Cancer. Breast Cancer. 2009;3:1-8.

298  Tang YM et al. Human CYP1B1 Leu432Val gene polymorphism: ethnic distribution African-Americans, Caucasians and Chinese: oestradiol hydroxylase activity; and distribution in prostate cancer cases and controls. Pharmacogenetics. Dec 2000;10(9):761-6.

299  O-leary P, Reddema P, Chan K, Taranto M, Smith M, Evans S. Salivary, but not serum or urinary levels of progesterone are elevated after topical application of progesterone cream to pre and postmenopausal women. Clin endocrinol. Nov 2000;53(5):615-20.

gesterone. Does that make urine testing invalid? Of course not! The different route of administration provides different metabolism and thus evaluation is different.

And did you also know that Weibe [300] has shown that some progesterone metabolites have a pro-growth potential (20-alpha and 2-alpha hydroxyprogesterone) and others have an anti-growth potential (5-alpha hydroxyprogesterone)? This has big implications in cancer. The impact of hormones is equally about hormone metabolism as it is about the individual levels and the balance themselves.

We are talking about men here and thus we need to look at testosterone. The testosterone metabolites include androsterone, Etiocholanolone, 5-alpha DHT, 5-beta DHT, 5-alpha Androstanediol, 5-beta Androstanediol, and Epi-testosterone. Most have never heard of these and the commercials definitely don't mention them.

Let's focus on the most important: 5-alpha DHT, 5-beta DHT, 5-alpha androstanediol and 5-beta androstanediol. Marketing would have you believe that testosterone is all there is. Testosterone is the end product. In reality, it is DHT. 5-alpha DHT is the active, most potent androgen (male hormone) and 5-beta DHT is inactive without androgenic activity. There is some suggestion that the 5-alpha androstanediol metabolite may be the better evaluative tool for 5-alpha DHT [301] [302]. In contrast, 5-beta DHT has a high

---

300  Wiebe JP. Progesterone metabolites in breast cancer. Endocrine-Related Cancer. 2006;13:717-738.

301  Frye CA, Edinger KL, Lephart ED, Walf AA. 3alpha-androstanediol but not testosterone, attenuates age-related decrements in cognitive, anxiety and depressive behavior in male rats. Front Agin Neurosci. Apr 8 2010;2:15.

302  Frye CA, Edinger KL, Seliga AM, Wawrzycki JM. 5-alpha-reduced androgens may have actions in the hippocampus to enhance cognitive performance of male rats. Psychoneuroendocrinology. Sep 2004;29(8):1019-27.

affinity for the estrogen receptor beta [303], which you will learn in the chapter on receptors why that is good. Notice that 5-alpha DHT and 5-alpha androstanediol are metabolites, but also biologically active.

Urinary metabolite testing is relatively new but its impact will be big.

## Saliva Testing

Saliva testing was the result of a desire to provide a better physiologic test. Saliva testing for hormones first appeared in the literature in the early 1980s. Saliva has become the medium of choice for many different reasons. First, saliva testing looks at the "free" hormone levels. A hormone has to be unbound from its carrier protein and free to elicit a physiologic action. So, saliva testing looks at the active hormone inside the cell at the site of action. That just happens to be the site of most of the receptors as well. Saliva testing has been validated for cortisol, estradiol, progesterone, DHEA, and testosterone [304] to name a few. Second, saliva testing requires no needles. That is right, if you have fear of needles you are in luck. Third, saliva testing has been shown to be well validated [305] and superior [306] than blood, with sensitivities and specificities exceeding 100% and 97.4% [307] respectively.

---

303  Picciarelli-Lima P et al. Effects of 3-beta-diol, an androgen metabolite with intrinsic estrogen-like effects, in modulating the aquaporin-9 expression in the rat efferent ductules.Reproductive Biology and Endocrinology. 2006;4:51.

304  Gavrilova N, Lindau ST. Salivary sex hormone measurement in a National, population-based study of adults. J. Gerontol B Pscychol Sci Soc Sci. Nov 2009;64B(suppl_1):i94-i105.

305  Nieman LK et al. The diagnosis of Cushing's syndrome: An endocrine society clinical practice guideline. JCEM. May 1 2008;93(5):1526-1540.

306  Perogamvros I, Owen LJ, Keevil BG, Brabant G, Trainer PJ. Measurement of salivary cortisol with liquid chromatography-tandem mass spectrometry in patients undergoing dynamic endocrine testing. Endocrinol (Oxf). Jan 2010;72(1):17-21.

307  Carrozza C et al. Clinical accuracy of midnight salivary cortisol measured by automated electrochemiluminescene immunoassay method in Cushing's syndrome. Annals of Clinical Biochemistry. May 2010;47(3):228-232.

Other than perfection, you can't get much better than that. And Fourth, according to the NIH (National Institute of Health), saliva testing will be useful in "detecting various cancers, heart disease, diabetes, periodontal disease..." [308]. From the functional/metabolic view, saliva testing is the best. No opinion, just scientific fact based on a summary of the scientific literature.

Saliva testing is also valid in disease evaluation. Saliva testing of cortisol has been recommended as the first-line test for Cushing's syndrome according to the endocrine Society's clinical practice guideline from 2008, due to "high diagnostic accuracy". A recent analysis found salivary cortisol superior to blood and urine in the diagnosis of Cushing's Syndrome [309]. Saliva testing is now considered the "gold standard" [310] for cortisol evaluation.

You cannot manage what you cannot measure. Fortunately, we can measure many different aspects of hormone function. The goal of any evaluative test should be to look at the body from a functional view.

No matter how hard some would like you to believe it, the body doesn't function in a linear manner.

The clinical relevance is what is important. Testing the hormones at the sight of action provides the best physiologic approach. Testing the hormone metabolites provides the next best approach. The evaluation of hormones in blood, hormones in transit, provides the least physiologic assessment. Each test provides an appropriate measure. The question is, does that measure provide

---

308  NIH. Salivary Diagnostics. Retrieved from http://report.nih.gov/nihfactsheets/ViewFactSheet.aspx?csid=65.

309  Sakihara S et al. Evaluation of plasma, salivary, and urinary cortisol levels for diagnosis of Cushing's Syndrome. Endocrine Journal. 2010;47(4):331-337.

310  Yaneva M et al. Midnight salivary cortisol for the initial diagnosis of Cushing's Syndrome of various causes. JCEM. July 1 2004;89(7):3345-3351.

insight into physiologic dysfunction? And, can an appropriate therapeutic intervention be under-taken to effect a change?

## Individual hormone levels

Contrary to most thought, hormones are not just about individual numbers. Hormones are a means of communication in the body. I am always amazed at the answers I get when I ask post-menopausal women if they still make hormones. Most will say no. It has been my experience that most of them are told this by their medical provider. Of course, the answer is yes. Men are never asked if they still make Testosterone after 50. The body must have these hormones to live and to survive (see addison's disease).

The first point of hormones is are they normal but what is normal? That discussion could go for days. For a simple answer, normal is defined as within the statistical reference range of normal. The top 2.5% and the bottom 2.5% are determined to be statistically abnormal and all other 95% are normal. If I used that logic with my kids, a 65 on a test would be considered statistically normal right? From my perspective and my child's that would not be the case. They were closer to failing than succeeding. And thus the limitations of this simple definition of normal. This approach may work for disease medicine, but it is not the best for functional medicine.

The data on low Testosterone in men is pretty clear. Low T in men is associated with an increased risk of all cause mortality [311] [312]. But even better, Testosterone therapy in those with low T was

---

311   Khaw KT et al. Endogenous testosterone and mortality due to all causes, cardio-vascular disease, and cancer in men. Circulation. 2007;116:2694-2701.

312   Araujo AB et al. Endogenous testosterone and mortality in men: a systematic review and meta-analysis. The Journal of Clinical Endocrinology Metabolism. Oct 1 2011;96(10):3007-3019.

found to be associated with a reduction in mortality [313] [314]. So, not only is low T associated with bad outcomes, but the resolution of low T has been shown to reduce the bad outcomes. The bad outcome here being mortality, and you can't get any worse than that.

A large percentage of conversation surrounding Testosterone is around its impact on the prostate. This is no different than the debate around Estrogen and the breast in women. Does Testosterone cause prostate disease? Does Testosterone cause Prostatitis? Does Testosterone cause Benign Prostate Hypertrophy (BPH)? Does Testosterone cause prostate cancer? All good questions. The answer to these questions is a resounding NO! If these statements were true, every 20 year old would have prostatitis, BPH, and prostate cancer. No study has shown that Testosterone causes the above prostate diseases [315] [316].

The key to understanding the above conclusion statement is understanding the individual hormones. Testosterone is not a static hormone. It is biologically dynamic. Testosterone interacts with the androgen receptors, Testosterone is converted to other hormones (DHT and Estradiol), and Testosterone is metabolized to its respective metabolites for elimination. It is what the body does with Testosterone, whether endogenous or exogenous, that negatively impacts the prostate.

---

313  Shores MM, Smith NL, Forsberg CW, Anawalt BD, Matsumoto AM. Testosterone treatment and mortality in men with low testosterone levels. The Journal of Clinical Endocrinology Metabolism. April 11 2012:jc.2011-2591.

314  Ohlsson C et al. High serum Testosterone is associated with reduced risk of cardiovascular events in elderly men: The MrOS (Osteoporotic fractures in men) study in Sweden. Journal of the American College of Cardiology. Oct 11 2011;58(16):1674-1681.

315  Bhasin S et al. Managing the risks of prostate disease during Testosteorne replacement therapy in older men: recommendations for a standardized monitoring plan. J Androl. 2003;24:299-311.

316  Morales A. Androgen replacement therapy and prostate safety. Eur Urol. 2002;41:113-120.

The conversion of Testosterone to Estradiol is the culprit in the transition from prostate health to prostate disease [317] [318]. The conversion of Testosterone to Estradiol, through high aromatase activity, has been shown to play a significant role in prostatitis [35] [319], BPH [320] [321], and prostate cancer [322] [323] [324] [325] [326]. This high Testosterone to Estradiol conversion has even been shown to be responsible for elevations in Prostate Specific Antigen (PSA) [327] [328].

317  Ellem SJ, Risbridger GP. Aromatase and regulating the estrogen:androgen ratio in the prostate gland. The Journal of Steroid Biochemistry and Molecular Biology. Feb 28 2010;118(4-5):246-251.

318  Risbridger GP, Ellem SJ, McPherson SJ. Estrogen action on the prostate gland: a critical mix of endocrine and paracrine signaling. J Mol Endocrinol. 2007;39:183-188.

319  Ellem SJ et al. Increased endogenous Estrogen synthesis leads to sequential induction of prostatic inflammation (prostatitis) and prostatic pre-malignancy. The American Journal of Pathology. Sept 2009;175(3):1187-1199.

320  Clement K M Ho et al. Oestrogen and benign prostatic hyperplasia: effects on stromal cell proliferation and local formation from androgen. J Endocrinol. June 1 2008;197:483-491.

321  Rohrmann S et al. Serum sex steroid hormones and lower urinary tract symptoms in Third National Health and Nutrition Examination Survey (NHANES III). Urology. Apr 2007;69(4):708-13.

322  Salonia A et al. Circulating Estradiol, but not Testosterone, is a significant predictor of high-grade prostate cancer in patients undergoing radical prostatectomy. Cancer. Nov 15 2011;117(22):5029-38.

323  Bonkhoff H, Berges R. The evolving role of Oestrogens and their receptors in the development and progression of prostate cancer. European Urology. Mar 2009;55(3):533-760.

324  Bosland MC. The role of Estrogens in prostate carcinogenesis: a rationale for chemoprevention. Rev Urol.2005;7(Suppl 3):4-10.

325  Carruba G. Estrogen and prostate cancer: An eclipsed truth in an androgen-dominanted scenario. Journal of Cellular Biochemistry. Nov 2007;102(4):899-911.

326  Giton F et al. Estrone sulfate (E1S), a prognosis marker for tumor aggressiveness in prostate cancer (PCa). The Journal of Steroid Biochemistry and Molecular Biology. Mar 2008;109(1-2):158-167.

327  Hill M et al. Analysis of Relations between serum levels of Epitestosterone, Estradiol, Testosterone, IGF-1 and Prostate Specific Antigen in men with Benign Prostatic Hyperplasia and Carcinoma of the Prostate. Physiol Res. 2000;49(Suppl 1):S113-S118.

328  Nakhla AM, Romas NA, Rosner W. Estradiol Activates the prostate androgen receptor and prostate-specific antigen secretion through the intermediacy of sex hormone-binding globulin. The Journal of Biological Chemistry. Mar 14 1997;272:6838-6841.

The negative impact of Estrogen on the prostate is through the increase in inflammatory signaling, and its interaction with Estrogen receptor alpha (ER alpha). Low Testosterone and high Estradiol production causes a shift from ER beta dominance to ER alpha dominance in the stoma of the prostate (read more about Estrogen receptors below and in chapter 9) . The interaction with the increased Estrogen production with the ER alpha promotes a more pro-inflammatory and pro-growth for the prostate. Not only does high Estrogen production promote inflammation, but high Estrogen production promotes a shift in ER dominance that favors an inflammatory translation.

## Hormone Balance

The second point on hormones is hormone balance. Balance is the source of health and wellness. Just look at our bodies. Our bodies are all about balance. Our bodies were created in balance– 2 eyes, 2 ears, 2 legs…Just trying losing a leg and see how the rest of your body is effected. You are likely to end up with bumps, bruises, and even worse. The loss of balance is often the precipitating cause of symptoms short term and disease development long-term.

Symptoms are the bodies attempt to get our attention and tell us that something is off balance. We must listen to our bodies. If we ignore our symptoms, or worse yet band-aid them, then we are fueling the fires of disease. But, if we use the symptoms to find the biochemical-physiologic imbalance, then the body can be healed.

Yes, you heard me right—healed. The body can be healed. If you focus on manging disease, that is all you will do. But focus on healing and you may just achieve it. How does the saying go, "you will never know what you can achieve until you try".

Hormones don't exist in a vacuum as many would have you believe. Hormones exist in a delicate balance. The most well publicized imbalance is that of the Estrogens and Progesterone in women. We are talking about endogenous hormones (synthetic hormones need not apply). Imbalance of Estrogen and Progesterone have been linked to many health problems: fatigue, weight gain, headaches, and increased risk of breast cancer in women–to name a few.

In men, the balance is less publicized. The major hormone balance in men is centered around Testosterone, DHT, and Estradiol. Testosterone is a prohormone. As a prohormone, Testosterone has biological activity, but it is either converted to Estradiol or Dihydrotestosterone and that is where the balance comes in to play. The balance between Estradiol and DHT is key. If the conversion to Estradiol dominates, through high aromatase activity, then low Testosterone results. The high Estradiol conversion inhibits Testosterone production through negative feedback at the level of the hypothalamus and the pituitary. Excess Estrogen in men is highly inflammatory as well. All the result of a low Testosterone:Estradiol balance. But if the enzyme 5-alpha reductase dominates, then Testosterone to DHT production dominates and the result is normal Testosterone:Estradiol balance. No feed back inhibition occurs, no proinflammation from excess Estrogen, and a normal Testosterone and DHT are the result.

But, there is another balance that I eluded too. The balance of aromatase and 5-alpha reductase. These are the enzymes that process Testosterone to either Estradiol or DHT respectively. Enzymes are proteins that move things along in our biochemistry. They convert product A to product B.

Aromatase is the enzyme that converts Testosterone to Estradiol. 5-alpha reductase is the enzyme that converts Testosterone to DHT. The balance of these two enzymes, aromatase:5-alpha reductase, helps to determine the balance between Testosterone:Estradiol, and DHT:Estradiol.

There are other balances equally important that are not discussed here: 5 alpha:5 beta reductase and Androstenedione:Estrone are two such examples.

I often tell clients that with every cause there is an effect. You can't give one hormone without it effecting many others. Testosterone is the perfect example. The addition of Testosterone, when low, may restore normal Testosterone levels. But in a majority of men today, it will increase Estradiol conversion (remember fat increases aromatase activity). This exaggerates the low Testosterone through feed back inhibition and promotes inflammation–all via estrogen. The balance of hormones allows one to see what the body will do with the hormones when hormone therapy is required. What does the body need and what is the body going to do with what it needs. A complete picture of hormones provides the safest picture for hormone therapy.

In men, Testosterone is usually the first treatment tried, when in fact, Testosterone should always be the last treatment for men with low T. The reason? Low Testosterone is usually the effect, not the cause. As I pointed out in chapter 4, there are diverse causes of low Testosterone: natural decline, stress, estrogen, obesity, inflammation, toxins, medications, and hormone therapy. The goal of all treatment should be a solution based therapy. Of course, we cannot effect aging (goes right along there with death and taxes). But, as a physician, we can effect change in stress, obesity, inflammation, toxins, medications, hormone therapy, and the biggest I see: Estrogen.

The presenting symptoms for most men that suggest low T are libido and ED. Face it, most men will run to their doctor's office due to a drop in libido, but concern for cardiovascular risk...well, not so much. What does the science say about libido and Testosterone. Very interesting data that point to the effects of Estrogen as the disruptor in sexual function, as described above, rather than Testosterone. Not a plethora of data here, but 3 studies point to high aromatase activity and resultant Estradiol and Estrone production in men with normal Testosterone and negatively effected libido [329] [330] [331]. Of course, when low T results, the symptoms significantly worsen. But, the symptoms appear to start with the respective causes.

How can high Estrogen and normal Testosterone levels result in physiologic effects like low libido and ED in men? The key may lie in the levels found in men [34]. Testosterone levels are measured in nanomoles, but Estrogen levels are measured in picomoles. One mole is equal to 1,000,000,000 nanomole compared to 1,000,000,000,000 picomoles. The laboratory effect is that higher Estrogen levels will be seen prior to a reflected change in Testosterone levels.

Not what you expected? Not what marketing says either. Just what the science says. Remember, it doesn't matter what marketing says, all that matters is physiology.

A couple of things to remember about libido–it is complex, even in men. This complexity accelerates in aging men due to altered hypothalamic-pituitary function, inflammation, altered androgen receptor sensitivity, and increased androgen protein binding (decrease free Testosterone) due to increase SHBG (Sex Hormone Binding Globulin) [332] [333] [334].

329  Knussmann R, Christiansen K, Couwenbergs C. Relations between sex hormone levels and sexual behavior in men. Arch Sex Behav. Oct 1986;15(5):429-45.

330  Phillips GB. Evidence for hyperoestrogenaemia as a risk factor for myocardial infarction in men. Lancet. July 3 1976;2(7975):14-8.

331  Goldmeier D, Scullard G, Kapembwa M, Lamba H, Frize G. Does increased aromatase activity in adipose fibroblasts cause low sexual desire in patients with HIV lipodystrophy? Sex Transm infect. 2002;78:64-66.

332  Taxel P et al. The effect of short-term treatment with micronized estradiol on bone turnover and gonadotrophins in older men. Endocr Res. Aug 2000;26(3):381-98.

333  Pugeat M et al. Clinical utility of sex hormone-binding globulin measurement. Horm Res. 1996;45(3-5):148-55.

334  Bancroft J. The endocrinology of sexual arousal. J. Endocrinol. Sept 1 2005;186:411-427.

For many men, the cause of low T is increased aromatase activity and Estrogen production. If we want to follow a solutions based therapy, then the first step would be to slow aromatase activity and see if Testosterone levels respond.

And the appropriate question would be: "has that been studied?" I am so glad you asked. The answer is yes. A 2004 study published in the prestigious *Journal of Clinical Endocrinology Metabolism*, looked at 37 "elderly men" (62-74 y/o). They treated these men with anastrazole, a synthetic aromatase inhibitor and drug commonly utilized in breast cancer. Their conclusion says it all: "These data demonstrate that aromatase inhibition increases serum bioavailable and total Testosterone levels to the youthful normal range in older men with mild hypogonadism" [335]. A second study was published in 2005 in *Clinical Endocrinology* and is essentially the same analysis, but looked to see if other variables were negatively effected. They were not. The conclusion is the same as the first: "... short-term administration of anastrozole is an effective method of normalizing serum Testosterone levels in elderly men..." [336]. But these two studies are looking at prescription anastrazole.

What about something natural? Something that you can do over the counter? And in this approach, we must make extra sure that the scientific data available supports it because it is a "natural" therapy. Unfortunately, natural therapies are considered guilty until proven otherwise by traditional medicine. So, research regarding any natural therapies must provide extra support. Not fair, but just the world we live in.

There are natural aromatase inhibitors. They are commonly known as bioflavonoids. Bioflavonoids are plant based antioxidants and

335 Leder BZ et al. Effects of Aromatase inhibition in elderly men with low or borderline-low serum testosterone levels. J Clin Endocrinol Metab. 2004 Mar;89(3):1174-80.

336 Dougherty RH et al. Effect of aromatase inhibition on lipids and inflammatory markers. Clin Endocrinol. 2005 Feb;26(2):228-35.

found extensively in plants [337]. The most effective and studied is the bioflavonoid chrysin [338] [339]. Chrysin is from the blue passion flower, or scientifically speaking: Passiflora caerulea. Chrysin is available over the counter, but the most effective form is through the skin in a transdermal cream. OTC chrysin commonly comes in pill form. A daily dosage of 500 to 1,000 mg would be common strategy for natural aromatase inhibition. The transdermal form can be found through your local compounding pharmacy by prescription. Dosages of 25-50 mg transdermal is the typical daily dosage. At these dosages, there are no concerns for any side effects.

So, is it possible that we can eat our chemotherapy? Is it possible that we can eat our aromatase inhibitors? Is it possible that, through diet, we men can limit the #1 cause of low Testostorone–high aromatase activity and increase Estrogen production? The questions are of course rhetorical. The answer is yes. Chrysin is the perfect example, as it is a flavonoid. Dietary sources of flavonoids include:

- berries (blueberries, cranberries, blackberries, cherries)
- grapes
- bananas
- grapefruit
- lemons
- limes
- oranges
- nuts (walnuts, pecans, and cashews)
- dark beans
- soybeans

337  Spencer, Jeremy PE. Flavonoids: modulators of brain function?" British Journal of Nutrition. 2008;99:ES60-77.

338  Jeong HJ, Shin YG, Kim IH, Pezzuto JM. Inhibition of aromatase activity by flavonoids. Arch Pharm Res. 1999 Jun;22(3):209-12.

339  Campbell DR, Kurzer MS. Flavonoid inhibition aromatase enzyme activity in human preadipocytes. J Ster Biochem and Mol Biol. Sept 93;46(3):381-88.

- red and green vegetables
- nightshade vegetables (peppers, tomatoes, and eggplant)

There are many natural sources of natural aromatase inhibitors. Many of which can be found in a well balanced, healthy diet. Who says diet has nothing to do with low T?

Additional bioflavonoid sources include the glorious coffee bean [340], Quercetin [341], Epicatechin [342] of the infamous green tea, and citrus flavonoid hesperetin [343]. But my favorite combination is red wine and its resveratrol [344][345] (but remember, not too much, because high alcohol consumption increases aromatase activity), and cocoa found in the wonderful dark chocolate [346]. These are all rich sources of bioflavonoids and thus natural aromatase inhibitors[347][348][349].

---

340 Osawa Y et al. Aromatase inhibitors in cigarette smoke, tobacco leaves and other plants. Enzyme Inhib. 1990;4(2):187-200.

341 Krazeisen A, Breitling R. Moller G, Adamski J. Phytoestrogens inhibit human 17beta-hydroxysteroid dehyrdogenase type 5. Mol Cell Endocrinol. Jan 22 2001;171(1-2):151-162.

342 Satoh k et al. Inhibition of aromatase activity by green tea extract catechins and their endocrinolgoical effect of oral administration in rats. Food Chem Toxicol. Jul 2002;40(7):925-33.

343 Ye L et al. The citrus flavonone hesperetin inhibits growth of aromatase expressing MCF-7 tumor in ovariectomized athymic mice. The Journal of Nutritional Biochemistry. Oct 1 2012;23(10):1230-1237.

344 Wang Yun et al. The red wine polyphenol resveratrol displays bilevel inhibition on aromatase in breast cancer cells. Toxicol Sci. July 2006;92(1):71-77.

345 Eng ET et al. Anti-aromatase chemicals in red wine. Annals of the New York Academy of Sciences. Jan 24 2006;963:239-246.

346 Balunas MJ, Su B, Brueggemeier RW, Kinghorn AD. Natural products as aromatase inhibitors. Anticancer Agents Med Chem. Aug 2008;8(6):646-682.

347 Nga Ta, Walle T. Aromatase inhibition by bioavailable methylated flavones. J of Steroid Biochemistry and Molecular Biology. Oct 2007;107(1-2):127-29.

348 YC Kao et al. Molecular basis of the inhibition of human aromatase (estrogen synthetase) by flavone and isoflavone phytoestrogens: A site directed mutagenesis study. Environmental Health Perspectives. Feb 1998;106(2):85-92.

349 Chen S, Kao YC, Laughton CA. Binding characteristics of aromatase inhibitors and phytoestrogens to human aromatase. J of Steroid Biochemistry and Molecular Biology. April 1997;61(3-6):107-115.

These natural aromatase inhibitors don't have to be taken in pill form. They can be simply enjoyed in a healthy balance diet. Simply have 1-2 cups of green tea or coffee daily. For those of you with a sweet tooth, eat one small square of dark cocoa daily. For those of you wine snobs out there have a glass of red wine each evening. Add in transdermal chrysin daily and you have a great natural multi-prong strategy to limit aromatase activity, Testosterone to Estrogen conversion, and maintain normal Testosterone levels. I know that this flies in the face of traditional medical dogma, but the science supports the above and it does not support traditional medical dogma as stated.

So why the heavy referencing? This is not a term paper–I know. But I and other proponents of natural therapies have been accused of unscientific recommendations. Or worse quakery. But without obvious basis. I merely want to show that natural therapies do in fact work. The science is bountiful for many, not bountiful for some, but present for all. The science is not overwhelmingly positive, but is positively favorable. One thing that we can't do is wipe away the 1,000s of years of anecdotal evidence and cultural uses of these products (which is presently done). Many merely flip these therapies away as "placebo effect". Placebo effect for 10 people over 1 month, maybe. But placebo effect of entire cultures for 1,000s of years–I think not.

How would you define quackery: to propose natural therapies to live healthy lives to prevent disease OR to malign and mislead on data present that shows natural therapies do provide health and disease benefits? I let you be the judge of that, but the science for "natural" therapies are there unquestionable! Be careful too not confuse opinion with science. Many today wave the banner of opinion as science.

As we saw above, aromatase inhibition is a great way to limit aromatase activity and thus limit Testosterone to Estrogen conversion.

What about other, just natural, ways to stimulate and/or support Testosterone production?

## Tribulus

From the plant Tribulus terrestris. This plant is commonly known as the "puncturevine" and is classified as a weed by many due to it's invasive tendencies. Tribulus is naturally found throughout the majority of the lower 48 states of the US, but prefers the more warm, temperate climates. Tribulus has been said to increase testosterone levels naturally [350] [351], improve erectile dysfunction [352], improve male libido, and has been used throughout history as an aphrodisiac [353] [354] in traditional Indian and Chinese medicine. Tribulus is thought to stimulate testosterone and sperm production through stimulation of Leutenizing Hormone (LH) and Follicular Stimulating Hormone (FSH) at the level of the pituitary [355].

The use of Tribulus, a natural bioflavonoid that increases Testosterone production, is well supported in the science. We established that in the previous paragraph. Now how to use it?–easy. Using the product that is mixed at 55:1 extract from Tribulus terrestris and protodioscin

350 Gauthaman K, Adaikan PG, Prasad RNV. Aphrodisiac properties of Tribulus Terrestris extract (Protodioscin) in normal and casatrated rats. J Dent. Nov 2008;36(11):900-6.

351 El-Tantawy WH, Temraz A, El-Gindi OD. Free serum testosterone level in male rats treated with Tribulus alatus extracts. J Ethnopharmacol. April 21 2006;105(1-2):255-62.

352 Gauthaman K, Ganesan A P. The hormonal effects of Tribulus terretris and its role in the management of male erectile dysfunction–an evaluation using primates, rabbit, and rat. Phytomedicine. Jan 2008;15(1-2):44-54.

353 Gauthaman K, Akakan PG, Prasad RNV. Aphrodisiac properties of Tribulus Terrestris extract (Protodioscin) in normal and castrated rats. Life Sci 2002;71:1385-96.

354 Gauthaman K, Adaikan PG. Effect of Tribulus on nicotinamide adenine dinucleotide phosphate-diaphorase activity and androgen receptors in rat brain. J Ethnopharmacol. Jan 4 2005;96(1-2):127-32.

355 Milanov S, Maleeva E, Taskov M. MBI: Medicobiologic information 1985;4:27.

(produced by Medi Herb), dose once to twice daily. Tribulus is one of my go to natural therapies for naturally supporting Testosterone production in both the young and old. I have seen this restore morning wake up calls with men in a matter of days, if you know what I mean.

## Epimedium species (Horny goat weed)

Epimedium Grandiflora extract is also know as horny goat weed. Go figure, that the "trade name" for Epimedium Grandiflora gives insight to it's use. Horny goat weed has been used by traditional chinese medicine for thousands of years for erectile dysfunction and as an aphrodisiac. Many call it an "unproven treatment". But in fact, there is science to support horny goat weeds positive male effect. It has positive erectile effects, positive blood flow effects (which of course what an erection is anyways), and anti-estrogen effects [356] [357] [358] [359]. It's primary role of action is believed to be through phosphodiesterase 5 inhibition [360]. This is the exact mechanism by which the popular prescription therapies for ED work.

## Tongkai Ali extract (Long Jack)

I mean, who came up with these names?–"long" Jack. Tongkai Ali extract, aka, Long Jack is a flowering plant/small tree indigenous to Indonesia and Malaysia. Another equator plant and a component of ancient Asian

356 Shindel AW, et al. Erectogenic and neurotrophic effects of icariin, a purified extract of horny goat weed (Epimedium spp.) in vitro and in vivo. J Sex Med. Apr 2010;7(4 Pt 1):1518-28.

357 Wu H, Lien EJ, Lien LL. Chemical and pharmacological investigations of Epimedium species: A survey. Progess in Drug Research. 2003;60:1-57.

358 Xin ZC et al. Effects of icariin on cGMP specifice PDE5 adn cAMP-specific PDE4 activities. Asian J Androl. 2003;5:15-8.

359 Ning H et al. Effects of icariin on phosophodiesterase-5 activity in vitro and cyclic guanosine monophosphate level in cavernous smooth muscle cells. Urology. 2006;68:1350-4.

360 Dell'Agli M et al. Potent inhibition of human Phosphodiesterase-5 by Icariin derivatives. J Nat Prod. 2008;71(9):1513-1517.

medicine. Again, there is something to a product, whether herb or other natural therapies, when large cultures have used these products for thousands of years. That is called the science of observation.

How does it work? Contrary to the Tribulus and Horny goat weed, its exact mechanism of action is unknown. Some have proposed that Long Jack reduces the SHBG (sex hormone binding globulin) levels, causing an effective increase in "free" Testosterone. But that is still just a theory.

There are benefits documented in the science. Some of the research was done in rats. From increased sexual arousal to increased sexually performance, Long Jack has shown benefits to sexually unaroused and under performing male rats. That makes me laugh, because how in the world does one know which male rat is "under aroused" and "under performing" [361] [362]. I just find humor in these scientific articles sometimes. But, from managing the effects of Low T [363] to sexual health [364], human benefit is found in the science for Long Jack as well.

## Kampo

Kampo is not a specific herb per se, but rather a paradigm of medicine that relies heavily on the uses of accupuncture and herbs. Kampo is found in traditional Japenese medicine that has its roots from traditional chinese medicine. Some have estimates

361 Zanoli P, Zavatti M, Montanarie C, Baraldi M. Influence of Eurycoma longifolia on the copulatory activity of sexually sluggish and impotent rats. J Ethnopharmacol. Nov 12 2009;126(2):308-13.

362 Rajeev B, Karim AA. Tongkat Ali (Eurycoma longifolia Jack): A review on its ethnobotany and pharmacological importance. Fitoterapia. Oct 2010;81(7):669-679.

363 M.I.B.M. Tambi, Imran MK, Henkel RR. Standardised water soluble extract of Eurycoma longifolia, Tongkat ali, as testosterone booster for managing men with late-onset hypogonadism? Andrologia 2012;44(sl):226-230.

364 Chye PH. Traditional Asian folklore medicines in sexual health. Indian J Urol. 2006;22(3):241-5.

of its origin dating back to the Han Dynasty in 200 BC. Herbs in Japanese Kampo are standardized and regulated as are many of the drugs/treatments in use today in the United States are. Kampo is a component of mainstream Japanese medicine. Seeing your Kampo practitioner in Japan, would be like seeing your internist in the US.

Kampo is subject to the same scientific research and rigor that "traditional" medicine is today. In the eyes of the Asian medical community, research in Kampo is on the same level as research one would find, on say, beta blockers for hypertension. Is there any research on Kampo and low T? That answer would be yes. Kampo has been shown to help men with low Testosterone. Specifically, Kampo therapy has been shown to help men with late-onset hypogonadism [365] [366]. Just a fancy medical way to say: "low Testosterone with advancing age". But late-onset hypogonadism sounds more scientific.

Other natural therapies said to support Testosterone levels in men are: selenium, zinc, vitamin E, CoQ10, Alpha Lipoic Acid, DHEA, and pregnenolone. Let's focus on the most scientifically supported.

Pregnenolone and DHEA are not supplements per se, but actually both are hormones. Pregnenolone is often referred to as the "mother" hormone as it is the hormone precursor for most other hormones. Pregnenolone is used to feed the production of other hormones. Pregnenolone is available from certain neutraceutical companies or by prescription from your local compounding pharmacy.

---

365  Amano T, Lmao T, Takemae K. Clinical efficacy of Japanese traditional herbal medicine (Kampo) in patients with late-onset hypogonadism. The Aging Male. 2010;13:166-73.

366  Tsujimura A et al. Change in cytokine levels after administration of saikokaryuukotsurboreit or testosterone in patients with symptoms of late-onset hypogonadism. The Aging Male. March 2011;14(1):76-81.

DHEA, also known as Dehydroepiandrosterone, has been sold OTC for a long time. DHEA is an androgen, male hormone, originating mostly from the adrenal glands. The more stable form is the sulfate form known as DHEA-S. The dosing sold OTC is in 25 mg increments. A male dosing would be in the range of 25-100 mg daily. This is not a female dosage (more like 5-10 mg daily). But be careful, because you can make Estrogens out of that DHEA. This is why it is so important to use hormones under the guidance of a knowledgeable practitioner.

Vitamin E is a commonly used supplement for men struggling with prostate problems. But, vitamin E also has benefit in men struggling with low Testosterone issues. Why? Because they are all just one in the same. Same problem manifested in a different organ. Vitamin E's activity is primarily through its anti-oxidant activity. Anti-oxidant therapy will reduce inflammation. Remember that inflammation is one of the causes of low T. Vitamin E has been shown to improve sperm motility [367] and function [368] in men. Vitamin E is best taken at levels of 300-600 mg by mouth. But, make sure you have your levels evaluated because you may need more or you may need less. Your needs are unique to you.

The last supplement we will highlight here is zinc. Most are aware of Zinc and it's impact on the immune system. But, zinc is a trace mineral necessary as a cofactor in many physiologic pathways. Deficiencies of zinc are known to increase aromatase activity [369] [370]. And with a 35.7% obesity rate, the pump is already primed

---

367   Suleiman SA et al. Lipid peroxidation and human sperm motility: protective role of vitamin E. J Androl. 1996;17:530-7.

368   Kessopoulou E et al. A double-blind randomized placebo cross-over controlled trial using the antioxidant vitamin E to treat reactive oxygen species associated male infertility. Fertil Steril. 1995;64:825-31.

369   Om AS, Chung KW. Dietary zinc deficiency alters 5 alpha-reduction and aromatization of testosterone and androgen and estrogen receptors in rat liver. J Nutr. Apr 1996;126(4):842-8.

370   Sapota A, Darago A, Taczalski J, Kilanowicz A. Disturbed homeostasis of zinc and other essential elements in the prostate gland dependent on the character of

with high aromatase activity. Throw low zinc in the mix and it is like throwing fuel on the fire. There we go again: it keeps coming back to that Testosterone to Estrogen conversion pathway. Zinc deficiency is easily corrected with zinc replacement. Have your zinc levels evaluated prior to supplementation, because you may not actually need it and too much of a good thing is not necessarily a great thing. Typical daily zinc dose is 20-25 mg.

## Hormone Metabolism

The next point I often make with our clients about hormones is hormone metabolism. How the body processes hormones (metabolism), is just as important as the individual hormone levels and the hormone balance themselves. Let's use Estrogen metabolism for example (but the same applies to all hormones). Estrogens can be metabolized 3 ways: 2-hydroxy Estrone, 4-hyroxy Estrone, and 16-alpha-hydroxy Estrone. For many years, the increased risk (breast and prostate cancer to name a few) was thought to be found in the 2:16-hydroxyestrogen ratio. It was thought that increased metabolism through the 2-OH pathway provided protection over that of the 16-OH pathway. This was also known as the Bradlow-Zoegler Hypothesis. This has however, proven to not to be the case [371] [372].

In contrast, it has long been known that the 4-hydroxy Estrone pathway provides a lot of the risk associated with Estrogen metabolism [373]. This pathway results in many dangerous metabolites (break down products) known as quinones. Many women with breast cancer and

pathological lesions. Biometals. 2009;22:1041-1049.

371  Arsian A A et al. Circulating estrogen metabolites and risk for breast cancer in premenopausal women. Cancer Epidemiol Biomarkers Prev. Aug 2009;18(8):2273-9.

372  Obi N, Vrieling A, Heinz J, Chang-Claude C. Estrogen metabolite ratio: Is the 2-hydroxyestrone to 16alpha-hydroxyestrone ratio predictive for breast cancer? Int J Womens Health. 2011;3:37-51.

373  Gaikwad GW et al. Urine biomarkers of risk in the molecular etiology of breast cancer. Breast Cancer. 2009;3:1-8.

men with prostate cancer don't take bioidentical (BHRT) Estrogen or synthetic Estrogen therapy. Their problem, as it relates to hormones, comes from endogenous hormone production, environmental xenoestrogens, and hormone metabolization. Their risk primarily occurs as a result of how their body processes their own endogenous hormones.

All is not lost in the battle against the toxic equinone metabolites. There are natural means to inhibit the formation of the toxic equinone estrogen metabolites. You may know them from a common saying from you mother: "eat your vegetables". Specifically, eat your cruciferous vegetables. These are vegetables of the likes of broccoli, cauliflower, cabbage, and brussel sprouts. So, maybe mom does know best. Your health begins with what you put in your mouth; or at least with regards to estrogen metabolism it does.

The benefits of the cruciferous vegetables are found in the presence of Diindolyl-methane (DIM) and Indole-3-carbinol (I3C). Indole-3-carbinol is the primary product of digestion of cruciferous vegetables by the enzyme myrosinase. Indole-3-carbinol can then join with itself to form Diindolyl-methane (DIM). Both have activity, but the majority of the activity appears to be found in the end product, ie. DIM [374].

You may have heard of these compounds as they are very popular supplements today. I3C is listed over 600 times in the scientific research engine pubmed. DIM comes in at 268. Not to shabby for "supplements". The majority of the research around these compounds is in regards to cancer treatment and cancer prevention.

The proposed benefit? Detoxification support. Detoxification is extensively covered in chapter 12, so I won't go into great detail

---

374  Bjeldanes LF, Kim JY, Grose KR, Bartholomew JC, Bradfield CA. Aromatic hydrocarbon responsiveness-receptor agonists generated from indole-3-carbinol in vitro and in vivo: comparisons with 2,3,7,8-tetrachlorodibenzo-p-dioxin. Proc Natl Acad Sci U S A. 1991;88(21):9543-9547.

here. Essentially, detoxification is the process of converting a compound, through a series of steps, to a more excretable compound to then eliminate it from the body. These compounds, toxins, can be both endogenous or exogenous in origin. I3C and DIM respectively, have been shown to increase phase I and phase II detoxification [375] [376] [377]. Stimulation of phase I, but particularily phase II, will limit the toxic equinone intermediate formation. See chapter 12 for a more detailed discussion of detoxification.

Is the science definitive? No. IT NEVER IS. But does it support the use of I3C and DIM? The answer to that question is yes. Some research has shown some negative effects from the use of these products. Likely (because physicians never evaluate these pathways), that is because the individuals detoxification pathways in question were not evaluated and one can assume that phase I was stimulated without adequate phase II stimulation. Trust me, you stimulate phase I and don't adequately support phase II, the person will not feel well at all. Equinone toxins are the result of phase I detoxification and inadequate phase II. One can see how if heavy stimulation of phase I without appropriate phase II stimulation can increase the toxin load and thus increase disease risk (in this case cancer) [378]. This is why I never guess with regards to a client's biochemical pathways. I evaluate

---

375  Bonnesen C, Eggleston IM, Hayes JD. Dietary indoles and isothiocynatates that are generated from cruciferous vegetables can both stimulat apoptosis and confer protection against DNA damage in human colon cell lines. Cancer Res. 2001;61(16:6120-6130.

376  Nho CW, Jeffery E. The synergistic upregulation of phase II detoxification enzymes by glucosinolate breadkown products in cruciferous vegetables. Toxicol Appl Pharacol. 2001;174(2):146-152.

377  Wallig MA, Kingston S, Staack R, Jefferey EH. Induction of rat pancreatic glutathione S-transferase and quinone reductase activities by a a mixture of glucosinolate breakdown derivatives found in brussels sprouts. food Chem Toxicol. 1998;36(5):365-373.

378  Baird WM, Hooven LA, Mahadevan B. Carcinogenic polycyclic aromatic hydrocarbon-DNA adducts and mechanism of action. Envriron Mol Mutagen. 2005;45(2-3):106-114.

the biochemical pathways through testing. You know what they say about assume?

What about dosing? There are plenty of commercially available products out there. But, most OTC recommendations under dose. With regards to diindolylmethane (DIM), 300 to 600 mg in divided daily dosing is a great range for adult dosing. And for I3C, the dosage I like to use is 200 to 400 mg daily. Understand that these are therapeutic dosing under the guidance of a physician. Detoxification should occur under the guidance of a physician due to reasons documented above.

Another very helpful compound in hormone metabolism is Calcium-D-glucarate [379]. Calcium-D-glucarate has shown benefits in hormone dependent cancers like prostate [380], breast [381] [382], and colon cancer [383]. In Estrogen metabolism, calcium-D-glucarate increases the elimination of Estrogen. It does this through an increase in glucuronidation in phase II detoxification [384] [385].

---

379   Alternative Medicine Review. Calcium-D-Glucarate. Vol 7, number 4. 2002. Found online at http://www.thorne.com/altmedrev/.fulltext/7/4/336.pdf.

380   Walaszek Z, Szemraj J, Narog M, et al. Metabolism, uptake, and excretion of a D-glucaric acid salt and its potential use in cancer prevention. Cancer Detect Prev. 1997;21:178-190.

381   Abou-Issa, Koolemans-Beynen A, Meredith TA, Webb TE. Antitumour synergism between non-toxic dietary combinations of isotretinoijn and glucarate. Eur J Cancer. 1992;28:784-788.

382   Webb Te, Abou-Issa H, Stromberg PC, et al. Mechanism of growth inhibition of mammary carcinomas by glucarate and the glucarate:retinoid comgination. Anticancer Res. 1993;13:2095-2100.

383   Yoshimi N, Walaszek Z, Mori H, et al. Inhibition of azoxymethan-induced rat colon carcinogenesis by potassium hydrogen D-glucarate. Int J Oncol. 2000.16:43-48.

384   Horton D, Walaszek Z. Conformations of the D-glucarolactones and D-glucaric acid in solution. Carbohydr Res. 1982;105:95-109.

385   Walaszek A, Hanausek-Walaszek M. D-glucaro-1,4-lactone: its excretion in the bile and urine and effect on biliary excretion of beta-glucuronidase after oral administration in rats. Hepatology. 1988;9:552-556.

Dosing of Calcium-D-glucarate is best in the range of 1,500 to 3,000 mg daily. Again, this should be under the guidance of a physician or other knowledgeable medical provider.

Of course, the discussion of the different supplements could go on and on. There is sulphorophane, there is NAC, Alpha lipoic acid.... I could go on forever, but I just have to draw the line somewhere.

But all that is about Estrogen. What about Testosterone?

Less is known about Testosterone metabolism when compared to Estrogen. But one aspect of Testosterone metabolism that we can discuss is related to the single nucleotide polymorphism (SNP) UGT2B17. This variance in genetic expression alters how Testosterone is metabolized by glucuronidation. This SNP is carried by an estimated 60% of asian men and these men have a reduced capacity to metabolize Testosterone through reduced type of detoxification called glucuronidation [386]. The result is higher levels of systemic Testosterone and lower levels of urinary Testosterone excretion. Thus, these Asian men have higher systemic Testosterone levels due to decreased metabolization of endogenous Testosterone production. A simple product of genetics.

The metabolism of Testosterone by men is known to slow with age [387]. This may be merely an effect of aging. However, remember this, because a little Testosterone will go a long way in older men due to a decreased metabolism of Testosterone. Another reason that all men, regardless of age, need to be treated as an individual.

---

386 Jakobsson J et al. Large differences in testosterone excretion in Korean and Swedish men are strongly associated with UDP-glucuronosy transferase 2B17 polymorphism. JCEM. Dec 6 2005;91(2):687-693.

387 Coviello AD et al. Differences in the apparent metabolic clearance rate of Testosterone in young and older men with Gonadotropin suppression receiving graded doses of Testosterone. The Journal of Clinical Endocrinology Metabolism. Nov 1 2006;91(11):4669-4675.

## Hormone Receptors

This is the one that gets most people. I focus on hormone receptors in chapter 9, but just a few things about hormone receptors here. Most people have heard of estrogen receptor/progesterone receptor (ER/PR) as it relates to breast cancer and even in prostate cancer. In these cancers, testing is done on the tumor itself to determine the ER/PR status. In breast and prostate cancers, ER+/PR+ cancers will better respond to hormone therapies. But, hormone receptors also play an important role in normal hormone function. It also happens to be the one we don't know a lot about nor do we have the capability to test in the clinical setting. But, just because we can not evaluate it, does not mean that it still doesn't play a role in function every second of every day.

Hormone receptors are just what they sound like. They are the receptors that the individual hormones bind too. Once the hormone binds to the receptor, the signal of the hormone is then internalized inside the cell through a series of secondary messengers. Most of these signals are genomic ie. interacting with the genes inside the nucleus of the cell. There are, however, non-genomic signaling that also occurs.

There is not just one receptor for each hormone. For example, with regards to estrogen, there are 2 different hormone receptors: alpha and beta. Which hormone receptor that is active and/or dominant determines the signal sent by the hormone. Think about this analogy: I have 4 children. If I tell each one of them to clean their room, I will undoubtably get 4 different responses. The message I deliver is the same, but the message is interpreted differently. For example, in the prostate in men, the ER alpha promotes inflammation, whereas ER beta does not promote inflammation. ER alpha promotes growth in the prostate in men. Vice versa, ER beta promotes apoptosis (cell death) and thus inhibits growth. The signal is the same–Estrogen. But, how the message is interpreted is completely opposite.

A little bit more about the Estrogen receptors. The body makes 3 types of estrogens: Estrone (E1), Estradiol (E2), and Estriol (E3). These Estrogens are not created equally. Their impact differs by the interpretation of the message through the Estrogen receptors. Estrone has been shown to increase breast cancer risk and prostate cancer risk. How? Estrone binds preferentially to ER alpha 3:1 compared to ER beta. So, Estrone increases inflammation and growth by a factor of 3:1 due to the receptor. In contrast, Estradiol binds to each receptor equally, 1:1. By contrast, Estriol has been shown to be beneficial in cancer. Why? I bet you know the answer. Estriol binds preferentially to the ER beta by a factor of 5:1. So, by a factor of 5:1, Estriol inhibits growth and reduces inflammation. All by the message interpretation through the receptors.

What about androgen receptors? Well, they are a little more limited. There is only one Testosterone receptor that we are aware of. Both Testosterone and DHT bind to the same receptor. DHT has a higher affinity for the androgen receptor than does Testosterone.

Low Testosterone in men has been shown to cause a change from ER beta (non-inflammatory) to ER alpha (inflammatory) expression in the male prostate. This move increases inflammation and plays a role in BPH and prostate cancer risk. Let me make this a little more clear: 35.7% of adults are obese according to 2011 CDC statistics. The increase in abdominal fat results in increased Testosterone to Estrogen conversion through aromatase activity. This high Estrogen concentration (low Testosterone to Estradiol ratio) feeds back to the hypothalamus and pituitary of the brain to inhibit the signaling that results in testicular Testosterone production. The result is low Testosterone. But, the low Testosterone state also changes the way the body responds to the Estrogen as well. The normal ER beta dominant state changes to an ER alpha state. This results in an inflammatory signal from the Estrogen. The impact–Inflammation, a pre-request for disease.

See how low Testosterone in men is more than just a gel or injection of Testosterone.

This is probably why hormone replacement in women, as they transition through menopause, provides many health benefits. But, when given in the postmenopausal state, many of those same health benefits go away and in fact turn negative. The body has, in fact, changed how it responds to the hormones. And as shown above, this also applies to men as well. But try to have this discussion with a physician whose go-to treatment for low T is Testosterone replacement. And if that doesn't work, then you just need more.

## Outside influences

We are all products of our genetics and our environment. That is called epigenetics. The same "environment" that influences our hormones, also influences the expression of our genetics.

There are many different environmental or outside influences on our hormones. I will focus on Xenoestrogens.

Xenoestrogens are environmental toxins that have Estrogenic activity. These are themselves toxins and disrupt biochemistry through that same mechanism. But, xenoestrogens also bind to Estrogen receptors and elicit Estrogenic activity. Remember, Estrogens inhibit Testosterone production.

These compounds include toxins such as parabens, Bisphenol-A (BPA), organophosphates, and pthalates to name a few. They all have been shown to elicit Estrogenic activity and thus be classified as xenoestrogens. You may have heard of them and you may not have. But, let me give you an example using the more commonly know Bisphenol-A (BPA).

A study was done on mice that were exposed to BPA. One group of male mice were exposed to BPA and a second group of male mice were not exposed to BPA. The male mice were placed in an environment with female mice and the female mice would not mate with the BPA exposed male mice [388]. So, maybe the reason a guy can't get a date has more to do with his BPA levels than his looks. Joking aside, this study showed that BPA exposure altered behavior, particularly sexual behavior.

But, it gets even better than that. Bisphenol-A has been shown to increase ER alpha expression. So, not only is Bisphenol-A a xenoestrogen [389], but at the same time, it changes the translation of the message to a more inflammatory, pro-growth message through the ER alpha[390] . Add in that BPA is an androgen receptor antagonist [391] and a thyroid receptor antagonist [392], directly decreases Testosterone via action at the testis [393] and pituitary [394],

---

388  Jasarevic E et al. Disruption of adult expression of sexually selected traits by developmental exposure to bisphenol A. Proc Natl Acad Sci U S A. Jul 12 2011;108(28).

389  Welshons WV, Nagel SC, vom Saal, FS. Large Effects from small exposures. III. Endocrine mechanisms mediating effects of Bisphenol A at levels of human exposure. Endocrinology. June 1 2006;147(6):s56-s69.

390  Richter CA et al. Estradiol and Bisphenol A stimulate androgen receptor and estrogen receptor gene expression in fetal mouse prostate mesenchyme cells. Environ Health Perspect. June 2007;115(6):902-908.

391  Lee HJ, Chattopadhyay S, Gong EY, Ahn RS, Lee K. Antiandrogenic effects of bisphenol A and nonylphenol on the function of androgen receptor. Toxicol Sci. Sep 2003;75(1):40-6.

392  Moriyama K et al. Thyroid hormone Action is disrupted by Bisphenol A as an antagonist. JCEM. Nov 1 2002;87(11):5185-5190.

393  N'Tumba-Byn T et al. Differential effects of Bisphenol A and diethylstilbestrol on human, rat and mouse fetal leydig cell function. PLoS ONE.7(12):e51579.

394  Nakamura D et al. Bisphenol A may cause testosterone reduction by adversely affecting both testis and pituitary systems similar to estradiol. Toxicology Letters. April 15 2010;194(1-2):16-25.

and potential links of BPA exposure to the increasing incidence of testicular cancer [395] and the picture of the damaging effects of BPA becomes crystal clear. The kicker is that the exposure of the pregnant mother to BPA and other xenoestrogens can kick start this hormonal dysfunction even prior to birth [396].

A very recent publication further highlighted the impact of Bisphenol-A on Testosterone. A study published in the prestigious Journal of Sterility and Fertility [397] found that serum Bisphenol-A was found to be statistically significant in it's association with low Testosterone and low Androstendione (weak androgen of adrenal origin). Also, an associated increase of SHBG was found, which makes logical sense, as Bisphenol-A is a xenoestrogen and Estrogens increase SHBG which will result in lowered free, available Testosterone.

And everybody just thought that men have low T and need Testosterone. When it comes to hormones, whether in men or women, the hormone levels are just the tip of the iceberg. The other hormone factors and metabolic function represent the mile of ice below the water. The tip of the iceberg is not what sank the titanic. The mile of ice below the water is what did the damage.

I realize that this chapter started off with the quote: "brevity is the soul of wit". But, there is a lot to say as it relates to hormones. A lot to say, as you can see, that is supported in the scientific literature.

---

395 Bouskine A et al. Estrogens promote human testicular germ cell cancer through a membrane-mediated activation of extracellular regulated kinase and protein kinase A. Endocrinology. Feb 2008;149(2):565-73.

396 Monje L, Varayoud J, Luque EH, Ramos JG. Neonatal exposure to bisphenol Amodifies the abundance of estrogen receptor alpha transcripts with alternative 5-untranslated regions in the femal rate preoptic area. J Endocrinol. Jul 1 2007;194:201-212.

397 Zhou Q et al. Serum bisphenol-A concentration and sex hormone levels in men. J Fertility and Sterility. May 6, 2013. doi:10.1016/j.fertnstert.2013.04.017.

# CHAPTER 9

# RECEPTORS

Perspective. It is amazing how different things can be when viewed from different perspectives. When I stand out in my back yard, I am wowed by God's creation. When I look out the window on my many plane flights, I am amazed by God's creation. But, when I see the perspective from space as seen by the astronauts...a whole new perspective on God's creation–awe-struck.

Perspective.

How accurate is your perspective? The more of the picture one can see the better the perspective. Perspective is very important when it comes to hormones.

If only men were just about Testosterone and women were just about Estrogen. Life would be easy and all would be symptom and disease free. That is the current perspective. But, it is not an accurate physiologic perspective. The body doesn't care about marketing: it only cares about physiology.

When it comes to hormones there are many components necessary for physiologic function and symptom free living.

**First**, the hormone levels need to be in the "normal" range: not too high, not too low. **Second**, the hormones need to be balanced. Women are more than Estrogen and men are more than Testosterone. **Third**, is hormone metabolism. We know, for example, that some of the risk associated with hormones is how the individual metabolizes, or better, detoxifies the hormones. **Fourth**, are outside micronutrients such as Magnesium and Zinc. Magnesium and Zinc are cofactors in the pathways of hormone production and metabolism. Low Magnesium and low Zinc levels can effect the normal function of hormones, despite normal hormone levels, normal hormone balance, and normal hormone metabolism. **Finally**, and the purpose of this chapter, are the receptors.

One almost never hears of the receptors role in proper hormone function. Receptors are how the signal is interpreted. That is the role of hormone receptors. The analogy I gave in chapter 8 on Hormones deserves repeating: I have 4 beautiful children. As with any parent, getting them to clean their room is an on going battle. When I ask them to clean their room, that is where the analogy is evident. The signal I give them is the same, clean your room, but how that signal is interpreted is quite different. And that signal may be interpreted differently dictated by the environment or pre-existing conditions. If my children are in one of their "moods", then they may just not clean their rooms out of defiance. How the signal is interpreted is just as important as the signal that is to be interpreted.

The greatest breakdown in any relationship is in communication. There is of course the words that are said. There is also the the way the words are interpreted. And then, there is the proper medium for conduction of the message. It takes all 3 variables: proper words, proper medium, and correct interpretation of words to provide good, effective communication. Hormones are no different. Hormones are a means of communication requiring proper interpretation for good hormone function.

What are hormone receptors? Scientifically speaking, hormone receptors are defined as: "a large family of ligand-activated nuclear transcription regulators, which are characterized by organization into different functional domains and are conserved, to differing degrees, between species and family members" [398].

But in plain language, hormone receptors are the medium the hormones use to communicate to the internal genome to turn genes off and on. There is also non-genomic signaling (hormone communication that does not effect DNA), but a large portion of signaling is with your DNA, also referred to as the classical pathway. That is what hormones do. They interact and turn off and on the expression of your DNA. Pretty amazing, huh? And you just thought that hormones floated through your blood causing hot flashes in women or ED in men. That is the way most, including physicians, see hormones today. That just couldn't be further from the truth.

Hormone receptors are in medical use today. Every person that has had or has been touched by someone with prostate or breast cancer is familiar with the term ER/PR positive or negative. This is in reference to Estrogen receptors and Progesterone receptors. This evaluation occurs from an actual tissue sample from the tumor itself and allows the medical team to determine the best course of action for that particular individual. In ER/PR positive tumors, hormone therapy is used; in contrast with ER/PR negative tumors, hormone therapy is not.

But what about those individuals who don't have cancer, but do have hormonal symptoms? Stay tuned. This testing hasn't made

---

398  Scarpin KM, Graham JD, Mote PA, Clarke CL. Progesterone action in human tissues: regulation by progesterone receptor (PR) isoform expression, nuclear positiong and coregulator expression. NURSA. 2009;7:1-13.

it to the clinical setting yet, but the results of animal testing holds great promise for the future in helping to complete the full picture and improve the perspective on hormones. Despite no current availability of testing in the non-tumor state, a thorough discussion of the scientific literature is required to complete the hormone picture.

So remember, don't kill the messenger. It may just be how the message is interpreted.

This chapter is a little technical. As one editor described it, "I felt like I was riding a rip stick while hanging onto a car traveling 70 miles an hour. This stroll through the minutia of the science of biochemistry is important to provide a thorough, accurate scientific discussion of hormones.

## Androgen Receptors (AR)

It appears that the androgen receptors are the easiest. I can here all the women reading this, "I could have told you that". Current knowledge is that there is just one androgen receptor (AR). These receptors are everywhere, but there is just one type. This receptor is encoded on the long arm of the X chromosome at position 12 [399]. That is just medical jargon for it is encoded on the X chromosome. The two most potent androgens, Testosterone and Dihydrotestosterone (DHT), both compete for this same receptor.

Testosterone is very important in development. But, what if I told you there was a more potent Testosterone? An androgen that inhibits Estrogen production. An androgen that is more potent. An androgen that does not get converted to Estrogens. An androgen

---

399  Tilley WD, Marcelli M, Wilson JD, McPhaul MJ. Characterization and expression of a cDNA encoding the human androgen receptor. Proc Natl Acad Sci U S A. Jan 1989;86(1):327-331.

that binds with a higher affinity and longer duration [400] (5 x longer) to the androgen receptor. That androgen is DHT. As stated in a 2000 publication of the Medical Journal of Australia [401]: "the varied actions of androgens in different tissues are not the result of distinct androgen receptors, but the result of the different levels of activity of aromatase and 5-alpha-reductase and therefore different relative levels of Testosterone, DHT, and Estrogens".

DHT is the most potent androgen with potency exceeding that of Testosterone by a ratio of 3:1 [402]. It's increased potency is through DHT's greater affinity for the androgen receptor. And that greater affinity is by a ratio of 3:1. As stated in the previous paragraph, DHT has a longer association time with the AR than does Testosterone. Testosterone compensates for this higher affinity and longer binding time by DHT, by increasing it's concentration relative to DHT. Only approximately 5% of Testosterone is converted to DHT. So, a smaller amount of androgen (DHT) has a larger signaling effect due to it's higher affinity and longer binding time with the androgen receptor. Also remember that there are 2 forms of the DHT–alpha and beta. The alpha-DHT is active and the beta-DHT is inactive.

Where are the androgen receptors? Are they just floating in the blood? Are they sitting on the surface of the cell just waiting for Testosterone or DHT to just come floating by? Just like a lazy saturday afternoon sitting on the porch watching cars drive by hoping someone stops to talk. Isn't that the visible picture given? It doesn't

400  Grino PB, Griffin JE, Wilson JD. Testosterone at high concentrations interacts with the human androgen receptor similarly to dihydrotestosterone. Endocrinology. Feb 1990;126(2):1165-72.

401  Handelsman DJ. Testosterone: use, misuse, and abuse. Med J Aust. 2006;185(8):436-439.

402  Wright AS et al. Relative potency of testosterone and dihydrotestosterone in preventing atrophy and apoptosis in the prostate of the castrated rat. J Clin Invest. Dec 1 1996;98(11):2558-2563.

matter what marketing says, it only matters what physiology is. Our physiology could really care less what we think–it works as designed or it does not.

The majority of androgen receptors are inside the cell. The interaction between Testosterone and DHT with the androgen receptors occurs in the cytosol of the cell. At that point the receptor under goes changes and then the signal is translocated to the DNA in the cell nucleus to turn DNA transcription on or off. But there is signaling via a non-genomic (non-DNA) pathway as well. This is why where you look to evaluate hormones is so important. If the hormone receptor interaction was in the blood, then look there–but it is not. If the interaction between the hormone and the receptor was in the urine, then look there–but mostly the metabolites are there; useful, but indirectly. But if you want to look at hormones at the sight of action, look at hormones in saliva. That shows you the free, bioactive hormone inside the cell. And where does the hormone interact with the receptor again? In the cell.

I don't want you to think that the androgen receptors are only inside the cell. That is actually referred to as the classical genomic pathway. Think interaction with the DNA when you think of the classical genomic pathway. But, there are also membrane androgen receptors that act via the non-classical genomic pathway. Then, there are pathways that don't appear to involve androgen receptors at all [403] [404]. Even within the receptors, there are variables. There are cytosolic AR and then there are membrane AR. There is classical genomic pathways and then there is non-classical pathways. There are pathways that use AR and those that don't use AR. The perspective on AR is complex.

---

403  Tep-areenan P, Kendall DA Randall MD. Testosterone-induced vasorelaxation in the rat mesenteric arterial bed is mediated predominantly via potassium channels. British Journal of Pharmacology. 2002;135;735-740.

404  Yue P, Chatterjee K, Beale C, Poole-Wilson PA Collins P. Testosterone relaxes rabbit coronary arteries and aorta. Circulation. 1995;91:1154-1160.

To see the importance of androgen receptors, look to what happens when they don't function well. Androgen receptor dysfunction has been implicated in "minor" disruption of male infertility [405] and decreased sperm production [406], to the complete disruption as in Androgen Insensitivity Syndrome (AIS). Androgen Insensitivity Syndrome is an individual that is genetically male, yet has the physical traits of a women–all because the male hormone message cannot be properly translated because of receptor dysfunction. Whether they be small genetic encoding errors (known as SNPs) or larger polymorphisms, the ability to properly interpret the hormone message is essential to proper function and health.

Testosterone and DHT have both been shown to decrease inflammatory signaling [407] [408]. The androgen receptors are anti-inflammatory as well. Androgen receptors are directly antagonistic to NFkappaB [409]. What is NFkappaB? NFkappB is a transcription factor that generates inflammatory signaling and androgen receptors antagonize this inflammatory signaling. It doesn't have to be the hormone that is anti-inflammatory, the androgen receptor itself can be anti-inflammatory. I will discuss more on inflammation in chapter 12.

---

405  Brinkmann, AO. "Androgen Physiology: Receptor and Metabolic Disorders." *Endotext.* N.p., Nov 2009.Web. www.endotext.org/male/male3/index.html.

406  Wang Ruey-Sheng et al. Androgen receptor roles in spermatogenesis and fertility: lessons from testicular cell-specific androgen receptor knockout mice. Endocr Rev. April 2009;30(2):119-132.

407  Hatakeyam H et al. Testosterone inhibits tumor necrosis factor-alpha-induced vascular cell adhesion molecule-1 expression in human aortic endothelial cells. 2002;FEBS Letters;530:129-132.

408  Vignozzi L et al. Antiinflammatory effect of androgen receptor activation in human benign prostatic hyperplasia cells. 2012. Journal of Endocrinology;214:31-43.

409  McKay LI, Cidlowski JA. Cross-talk between nuclear factor-kB and the steroid hormone receptors: mechanisms of mutual antagonism. Molecular Endocrinology. 1998;12:45-46.

## Estrogen Receptors (ER)

Then there was 2. Think things were complex with androgen receptors? Things really get complex when we get into Estrogen receptors. To be fair to the men in the audience, I can here their collective: "I could have told you that..."

Current understanding is that there are 2 Estrogen receptors: alpha and beta. These two different Estrogen receptor types appear to have some tissue specific expression [410] and can produce profoundly different results. Estrogen receptor alpha (ER alpha) has been found to be present in endometrium (lining of the uterus), breast, ovary, prostate, and hypothalamus. Conversely, Estrogen receptor beta (ER beta) has been found in kidney, brain, prostate, skeletal, and endothelial cells [411]. However, it is felt that Estrogen receptors are ubiquitously present in the body with tissue preference to the alpha and beta form.

Estrogen receptors are primarily located intracellularly (inside the cell). These receptors are particularly in the cytosol of the cell. The binding of Estrogen to the individual receptors then triggers a transformation in the receptor. The altered receptor then transports the signal to the nucleus of the cell. That has been the primary thought on Estrogen receptors for some time now. But, we now know that there are estrogen related receptors (discussed below) and we know that there are Estrogen receptors on the plasma membrane as well [412]. These membrane Estrogen receptors have been primarily studied and discussed in research on brain synapsis. These membrane Estrogen receptors originate from the same place as the intracellular receptors and appear to respond to a more localized Estrogen

---

410  Mueller SO, Korach KS. Estrogen receptors and endocrine disease: lessons from estrogen receptor knockout mice. Curr Opin Pharmacol. Dec 2001;1(6):613-9.

411  Koehler KF, Helguero LA, Haldose'n LA, Warner M, Gustafsson JA. Reflections on the discovery and significance of estrogen receptor-b. Endocrine Reviews 2005;26(3):465-478.

412  MacLusky NJ. Understanding the direct synaptic effects of estradiol. Endocrinology. Feb 2013;154(2):581.

production [413]. The more we learn, the more we discover we don't know.

As it relates to a lot of disease, ER-alpha has been shown to produce a more pro-inflammatory [414] and pro-growth [415] signal from Estrogen. Inflammation is a prerequisite for disease generation. Cancer requires inflammation and is simply unregulated growth. One cannot say all ER-alpha expression is associated with disease, but the scientific literature does favor a more disease generating environment with regards to ER-alpha dominant signaling. One can see how an ER-alpha dominant signal can favor disease generation with it favoring growth and inflammation. ER-alpha has been shown to play roles in breast cancer [416] , ovarian cancer [417], and prostate cancer [418] to name a few.

Contrast this with ER-beta. Estrogen receptor beta has been shown to produce a more anti-inflammatory [419] and anti-growth [420] sig-

413  Tabatadze N, Smejkalova T, Woolley CS. Distrubution and posttranslational modification of synaptic ERalpha in the adult female rat hippocampus. Feb 2013;154(2):819.

414  Vegeto E et al. Estrogen Receptor-alpha as a drug target candidate for preventing lung inflammation. Endocrinology. Jan 2010;151(1):174-184.

415  Ellison-Zelski SJ, Alarid ET. Maximum growth and survival of estrogen receptor positive breast cancer cells requires the Sin3A transcriptional repressor. Molecular Cancer. 2010;9:263.

416  Ali S, Coombes RC. Estrogen receptor alpha in human breast cancer: occurrence and significance. J Mammary Gland Biol Neoplasia. Jul 2000;5(3):271-81.

417  Chu S, Mamers P, Burger HG, Fuller PJ. Estrogen receptor isoform gene expression in ovarian stromal and epithelial tumors. J Clin Endocrinol Metab. 2000;85:1200-1205.

418  Ricke WA et al. Prostatic hormonal carcinogenesis is mediated by in situ estrogen production and estrogen receptor alpha signaling. The FASEB Journal. May 2008;22(5):1512-1520.

419  Catley MC et al. Estrogen Receptor Beta: expression profile and possible anti-inflammatory role in disease. JPET. July 2008;326(1):83-88.

420  Zhang J, Tu Y, Smith-Schneider S. Activation of p53, inhibition of telomerase activity and induction of estrogen receptor beta are associated with the anti-growth effects of combination of ovarian hormoens and retinoids in immortalized human mammary epithelial cells. Cancer Cell Int. Mar 8 2005;5(1):6.

nal from Estrogen. ER-beta has been shown to benefit asthma [16], prostate cancer [421], breast cancer [422], colon cancer [423] and even the excitotoxic diseases [424] : MS, Parkinson's disease, Alzheimer's, and ALS. It doesn't take a rocket scientist to see the potential positive impact of ER-beta. The anti-inflammatory and anti-growth activity of ER beta can be translated to more healthy and disease free living.

But does ER-alpha always produce a pro-inflammatory signal? Does ER-beta always produce a anti-growth response? Are these receptors tissue specific? Can the expression of ER-alpha and ER-beta change? These are some of the questions that have yet to be answered.

What the science does tell us, is that Estrogen receptors can change. Maybe this can explain some of the variation in hormone response between individuals? Or maybe this can explain the response difference in women to Hormone Replacement Therapy (HRT) in the years of peri-menopause versus that post-menopause. The Perfect example, is actually found in men. Men with low Testosterone are shown to have a shift from ER-beta to ER-alpha [425] dominance in the prostate. Now let's think about that for a moment. One of the primary causes of low Testosterone can be the result of increased Testosterone to Estrogen production from high aromatase activity. This is called Estrogen dominance–a term coined by John Lee. So

---

421   Weihua Z et al. A role for estrogen receptor Beta in the regulation of growth of the ventral prostate. Proc Natl Acad Sci U S A. May 22 2001;98(11):6330-6335.

422   Lazennec G et al. ERbeta inhibits proliferation and invasion of breast cancer cells. Endocrinology. Sept 1 2001;142(9):4120-4130.

423   Foley EF, Jazaeri AA, Shupnik MA, Jazaeri O, Rice LW. Selective loss of estrogen receptor beta in malignant human colon. Cancer Res. 2000;60:245-248.

424   Tiwari-Woodruff S, Morales LB, Lee R, Voskuhl RR. Differential neuroprotective and antiinflammatory effects of estrogen receptor (ER)alpha and ERbeta ligand treatment. Proc Natl Acad Sci U S A. Sep 11 2007;104(37):14813-8.

425   Cohen PG. Obesity in men: the hypogonadal-estrogen receptor relationship and its effect on glucose homeostasis. Med Hypotheses. 2008;70(2):358-60.

high Testosterone to Estrogen production causes low Testosterone. Men with low Testosterone have a shift from ER-beta to ER-alpha dominance. ER-alpha produces a pro-inflammatory and a pro-growth signal. Inflammation up-regulates aromatase activity. And did I mention that the cause of low T in many men is a high conversion of Testosterone to Estrogen? Which then is interpreted in a more pro-inflammatory and pro-growth manner. Vicious cycle?! This is why ER-alpha has been found to be associated with BPH and prostate cancer in men and breast cancer in women.

Additionally, the loss of ER-beta expression has been shown to increase prostate disease. In a recent study in mice, zero ER-beta was found to increase abnormal prostate cell growth (hyperplasia) [426]. Another study in mice, found ER-beta to stimulate decrease in prostate size and trigger cell death through apoptosis (programmed cell death) [427]. But we are talking about humans here. In human studies, ER-beta expression has been shown to reduce the incidence of prostate disease [428] [429]. Looks pretty promising that ER-beta expression in the male prostate is protective against prostate disease. But remember, low T induces a change from ER beta dominance to ER alpha dominance.

Just to stir things up a little more and show the complexity that really exists in hormones, let's look at Estrogen Related Receptors (ERR).

---

426 Imamov O et al. Estrogen receptor beta regulates epithelial cellular differentiation in the mouse ventral prostate. Proc Natl Acad Sci U S A. 2004;101:9375-9380.

427 Krishnana G et al. Novel ER beta selective agonists induce prostate atrophy in rodents without affecting the hypothalamo-pituitary-gonadal axis. In the Endocrine Society Annual Meeting 2004. 2004. The Endocrine Society Press. Chase, Maryland, USA. 180-181.

428 Leav I et al. Comparative studies of the estrogen receptors beta and alpha and the androgen receptor in normal human prostate glands, dysplasia, and in primary and metastatic carcinoma. Am J Pathol. 2001;159:79-92.

429 Horvath LG et al. Frequent loss of estrogen receptor-beta expression in prostate cancer. Cancer Res. 2001;61:5331-5335.

They exist in alpha, beta, and gamma forms [430]. These receptors are nuclear receptors just like regular Estrogen receptors. Estrogen related receptors have significant similarity to Estrogen receptors. But, they do not respond to Estrogen as do Estrogen receptors [431] [432]. The exact specific substrates (substances acted upon by an enzyme) for the Estrogen related receptors are yet to be determined. Estrogen related receptors are often referred to as "orphan" members of the nuclear receptor family [433]. Estrogen receptors are also a members of the nuclear receptor family. There has been question if there actually are any specific substrates for Estrogen related receptors and maybe these Estrogen related receptors just play an accessory role. However, they do bind Estrogen related elements. Estrogen related elements are just as they say—elements related to Estrogen, but not actual Estrogen. Nice, huh? The perfect example here is aromatase. Aromatase is the enzyme that converts Testosterone to Estradiol, yet it is not an Estrogen. However, aromatase makes Estrogen, and thus aromatase in this example is an Estrogen related element. What exact role these play in the overall hormone symphony? That is yet to be determined. But they definitely play a role.

Complex, huh? I hope that you see that hormones are more than just Estrogen or Testosterone and whether their levels are low or high. In fact, many clients I have seen have been told that they do

---

430   Coward P, Lee D, Hull MV, Lehmann JM. 4-Hydroxytamoxifen binds to and deactivates the estrogen-related receptor gamma. Proc Natl Acad Sci U S A. July 17 2001;98(15):8880-8884.

431   Heard DJ, Norby PL, Holloway J, Vissing H. Human ERRgamma, a third member of the estrogen receptor-related receptor (ERR) subfamily of orphan nuclear receptors: tissue-specific isoforms are expressed during development and in the audit. Mol Endocrinol. Mar 2000;14(3):382-92.

432   Vanacker JM. Pettersson K, Gustafsson JA, Laudet V. Transcriptional targets shared by estrogen receptor-related receptors (ERRs) and estrogen receptor (ER) alpha, but not by ER beta. EMBO J. Aug 2 1999;18(15):4270-4279.

433   Enmark E, Gustafsson J A. Orphan nuclear receptors: the first eight years. Mol Endocrinol. 1996;10:1293-1307.

not need their hormones evaluated prior to initiating therapy. I hope you can see the folly of that statement.

I believe hormone receptors to be the next great frontier in the arena of hormones. Hormones and hormone receptor interactions are complex and much is left to be learned. Hormones are simply not just about Estrogen for women and Testosterone for men. Not surprisingly, they are complex and unique to the individual.

The majority of the current research around Estrogen receptors is with breast and prostate cancer. However, the Estrogen receptors are ubiquitous in the body and play a significant role in normal physiology [434]. Eventually, Estrogen receptor testing will reach the clinical setting. Time will tell when. The more we learn about hormones the more we realize we don't know.

## Progesterone Receptors (PR)

And what of Progesterone receptors. Since progesterone is the hormone often excluded from consideration by traditional medicine, I figured it would be appropriate to leave it for last.

It has always amazed me, that prior to a hysterectomy women need Estrogen, Progesterone, and Testosterone (and other hormones) in balance for a normal cycle. But post hysterectomy, all women need is Estrogen. Hmmm? That thinking falls into the "all a woman is, is a uterus" mentality.

Please note, that the vast majority of the studies on Progesterone receptors are with regards to women. I still think it is important to discuss them here for the purpose of a comprehensive discussion of receptors.

---

434 Dickson RB, Stancel GM. Chapter 8: Estrogen receptor-mediated processes in normal and cancer cells. J Natl Cancer Inst Monogr. 2000;27:135-145.

Current understanding is that there are 3 Progesterone receptors (PR): A, B, and C. Progesterone receptors are nuclear receptors. That is right. Progesterone must enter the target cell and bind to the nuclear transcription factor to relay its message–just like the Estrogen and androgen receptor(s). The Progesterone:Progesterone receptor complex is then translocated to the DNA to effect DNA transcription. Transcription is the first step in reading the message from the DNA. From there it will be translated into mRNA and then into the final product form–like a protein. Progesterone receptors also regulate non-genomic (non-DNA) signaling as well.

The point here is not about transcription or translation, which are important, but that these receptors are in the nucleus of the cell. This is the reason that appropriate testing is so important. Testing must occur at the site of action (or at least as close as possible). It is much more clinically useful to evaluated the hormones inside the cell at the site of action (Progesterone receptor), than in the blood at no sight of action. That is why saliva testing is one of the better ways to evaluate many hormones. Saliva testing allows one to see Progesterone inside the cell at the site of the Progesterone receptors. In the blood, we have no idea of knowing whether the Progesterone is coming, going, or just along for the ride. Like the FedEx truck analogy I have used previously. You can have 100 FedEx trucks drive by your house, but if none stop, there is no delivery. That analogy holds for blood hormone evaluation.

PR-A and PR-B are the old kids on the block. They have been around the longest (at least known since the 1970s)[435] and appear to be the major isoforms of the Progesterone receptor. Progesterone receptors appear to be ubiquitously expressed in most tissue. The dominant expression of PR-A or PR-B likely explains the differing effects of progesterone in different target tissues. Even though Progesterone

---

435  Conneely OM et al. Reproductive functions of progesterone receptors. Recent Prog Horm Res. 2002;57:339-55.

receptors have been shown to be relatively equally expressed, PR-A and PR-B have been shown to have some tissue specificity. For example mouse studies have shown that PR-B is required for normal breast development [436] . Maybe the dominant Progesterone receptor present in breast tissue has more to do with the normal vs abnormal development of breast cells; versus the mere presence of Progesterone. As the old saying goes–"don't kill the messenger". The messenger is Progesterone. Don't kill the messenger! The problem could be just how the message is interpreted–the receptor.

Contrast this with PR-A, which has been shown to be required for proper development of the uterus and the proper functioning of the reproductive system [437] . These are just some examples of tissue specificity of the Progesterone receptors.

Progesterone receptor A is merely a shortened form [438] of Progesterone receptor B. Progesterone receptor A has been suggested to be the weaker [439] of the two receptors. However, Progesterone receptor A has been shown to be the primary inhibitor [440] of Progesterone receptor B. Contrast this with PR-B acting as a primary potent activator [441] of gene transcription (beginning

436  BMulac-Jericevic B et al. Defective mammary gland morphogenesis in mice lacking the progesterone receptor B isoform. Proc Natl Acad Sci U S A. Aug 19 2003;100(17):9744-9749.

437  Mulac-Jericevic B et al. Subgroup of reproductive functions of progesterone mediated by progesterone receptor-B isoform. Science. Sep 8 2000;289(5485):1751-4.

438  Gao X, Nawaz Z. Progesterone receptors-animal models and cell signaling in breast cancer: role of steroid receptor coactivators an corepressors of progesterone receptors in breast cancer. Breast Cancer Res. 2002;4:182-186.

439  Vegeto E et al. Human progesterone receptor A form is a cell- and promoter-specific repressor of human progesterone receptor B function. Mol Endocrinol Oct 1993;7(10):1244-55.

440  Tung L et al. Antagonist-occupied progesterone B-receptors activate transcription without binding to progesterone response elements and are dominantly inhibited by A-receptors. Mol Endocrinol. Oct 1993;7(10):1256-65.

441  Giagrande PH, Pollio G, McDonnell DP. Mapping and characterization of the functional domains responsible for the differential activity of the A and B isoforms

of gene signaling) of PR-A. So, even though the two PR isoforms are co-expressed, they effect the expression of the other.

Remember, don't kill the messenger.

The impact of the loss of Progesterone receptor balance is evident in disease [442]. It is when the co-expression of PR-A and PR-B on breast tissue [443] is lost, that cancer progression begins. In fact, the balance of PR-A:PR-B [444] (high PR-A expression) has been shown to effect survival rates in those with ER+/PR+ disease on hormonal therapy. The impact of PR doesn't stop with breast cancer. Abnormal cell growth in endometrial tissue (lining of the uterus) begins when the balance of PR-A and PR-B is lost [445]. The point is, that if the Progesterone receptor balance can effect disease progression and survivability, then Progesterone receptor balance can absolutely be involved in disease initiation and thus a better understanding of Progesterone receptor balance can be utilized for health and wellness for disease prevention in the future.

Less is known of Progesterone receptor isoform C. Progesterone receptor C (PR-C) is a shortened form of the dominant Progesterone receptors A and B. Progesterone receptor C appears to be a co-regulator of PR-A and PR-B [446]. Meaning? Progesterone receptor C

of the human progesterone receptor. J Biol Chem. Dec 26 1997;272(52):32889-900.

442  Scarpin KM, Graham JD, Mote PA, Clarke CL. Progesterone action in human tissues: regulation by progesterone receptor (PR) isoform expression nuclear positioning and coregulator expression. Nuclear Receptor Signaling. 2009;7:e009.

443  Mote PA, Bartow S, Tran N, Clarke CL. Loss of co-ordinate expression of progesterone receptors A and B is an early event in breast carcinogenesis. Breast Cancer Res Treat. Mar 2002;72(2):163-72.

444  Hopp TA et al. Breast cancer patients with progesterone receptor PR-A-rich tumors have poorer disease-free survival rates. Clin Cancer Res. April 15 2004;10:2751.

445  Arnett-Mansfield RL et al. Relative expression of progesterone receptors A and B in endometrioid cancers of the endometrium. Cancer Res. Jun 1 2001;61:4576.

446  Wei LL, Norris BM, Baker CJ. An N-terminally truncated third progesterone receptor protein, PR0C), forms heterodimers with PR(B) but interferes in PR(B)-DNA binding. J Steroid Biochem Mol Biol. Jul 1997;62(4):287-97.

is not the main activator or inhibitor of gene transcription (signaling), PR-C is just a necessary co-signal that enhances the primary receptors. Though it is not the primary route of signal transduction, it is still necessary.

Magnesium and Zinc that are cofactors in the pathways of hormone production and metabolism. Low Magnesium and Zinc levels can effect the normal function of hormones, despite normal hormone levels, normal hormone balance, and normal hormone metabolism.

It doesn't end there. It doesn't just end with the individual androgen, Estrogen, and Progesterone receptors. Balance of hormone receptors is just as important as the individual hormones. As with hormones, receptors effect each other. Just as to much Estrogen or to much Testosterone can create imbalance and effect other hormones, so can the receptors. Hormones don't exist in a vacuum; likewise hormone receptors don't exist in a vacuum.

This brings me back to the point that all hormones must be present and accounted for, not just Testosterone and Estrogen. It appears, based on the scientific literature, that the same must apply to the receptors for the hormones as well.

The different hormone receptor subgroups effect each other. It seems there is always another deeper step to take. Let's take that step to display the complexity of hormone receptors. Progesterone receptor A has been shown to decrease the efficacy of the Estrogen receptors (ER) [447]. It has been shown that the 2 forms of estrogen receptors (ER alpha and ER beta) can effect the transcription and expression of each other [448]. Thyroid hormone receptors have been shown to effect

---

447  McDonnell DP, Goldsman ME. RU486 exerts antiestrogenic activities through a novel progesterone receptor A form-mediated mechanism. J Biol Chem. April 22 1994;269:11945-11949.

448  Young LJ, Wang Z, Donaldson R, Rissman EF. Estrogen receptor alpha is essentital for induction of oxytocin receptor by estrogen. Nueroreport. 1998.9:933-926.

expression of Estrogen receptors. Estrogen receptors have been shown to effect the expression of thyroid receptors [46]. The balance of hormones extends to the receptors as well as to the hormones.

Hormone receptors are communicating and/or influencing the expression of the other hormone receptors. Not only can the messages influence each other (hormones), but how the messages are interpreted (hormone receptors) can influence each other. This can then turn around and influence the messages (hormones) themselves. Headache yet?

Do you see how the current medical model today just flat out misses the boat on hormones. Remember, the Institute of Medicine found that the average physician practices 17 years behind the current scientific knowledge. As I have said earlier: "It doesn't matter what marketing is or what doctors say, what matters is physiology". The body could care less about what I, any other medical provider, or marketing company thinks. It functions as the creator created it–beautifully complex. Men, you are much more than just a Testosterone fueled erection. You are more than just a product of Testosterone and DHT. You are a product of the androgens interaction with the androgen receptors and the genetic and non-genetic signaling that results. But of course, we are so much more.

# CHAPTER 10

# ENVIRONMENT

What role does the environment play in what amounts to a life and death drama? Does the environment directly affect hormones? The hormone messaging? The message interpretation? Does it affect the balance of the message? The volume of message? The interpretation of the message? Or is it all the above?

The answer is all the above.

The environment has changed and the changing environment is changing us. The perfect example of what a change in environment can do is present in a 1998 study on testosterone. This study found that Chinese men living in the US had lower testosterone levels than their counterparts living in China [449]. The conclusion says it all: "In conclusion, dietary or environmental factors, and not the diminution of 5alpha-reductase, appear to be responsible for differences in androgen metabolism between caucasians living in the United States and Chinese living in China". Similar genetic make up (Chinese) in a

---

449  Santner SJ et al. Comparative rates of androgen production and metabolism in caucasian and chinese subjects. The Journal of Clinical Endocrinology Metabolism. June 1 1998;83(6):2104-2109.

different environment (China versus US) produces different results. This same result has been found in breast cancer in women as well [450].

When it comes to health, the environment is an equal opportunity offender. Another 1993 Journal of National Cancer Institute study revealed a 60% increased risk of breast cancer in Asian-American women born in the western countries/cultures versus those born in the eastern countries/cultures [451]. Clearly, the environment is playing a role in our health today. To deny the association is to deny reality.

The use of the term "environment" can create a lot of confusion these days. Environment can elude to the "global warming" or "climate change" debate, which is not the case here. With respect to environment in this discussion, I am referencing the toxins that arise from the environment. These are toxins such as chemicals found in insecticides, pesticides, and plastics. Toxins don't just result from the environment, some are endogenous. Even our own bodies can produce toxins from normal physiologic metabolism. But here, I am discussing the impact of environmental toxins on hormone receptors. And the impact is significant, though hotly debated.

Unfortunately, politics have hijacked the term "environmental". It seems that if you are a Democrat, then everything is the result of environmental toxins (ie. organophosphates, organochlorides, Bisphenol A, etc). But if you are a Republican, there is no such thing as environmental toxins. It is one extreme or the other, with no in between. Politics! Ideology induced blindness on both sides. As we all know, politics doesn't equate to truth. In fact, the opposite is usually true.

---

450   Gomez SL et al. Hidden Breast Cancer disparities in Asian Women: Disaggregating Incidence rates by Ethnicity and Migrant Status. Am J Public Health. April 2010;100(Suppl 1):S125-S131.

451   Ziegler RG. Migration patterns and breast cancer risk in Asian-American Women. JNCI J Natl Cancer Inst. 1993;85(22):1819-1827.

Neither argument is accurate. Scientifically, the truth is that environmental toxins are playing a role in the health problems that we see today (just review the 2 studies listed two paragraphs above). Politics has, however, hijacked the science supporting the truth. No longer does truth drive politics, but politics steals truth to support ideology, irregardless of truth. Politics corrupts truth. Politics corrupts science.

An excellent example of politics clouding the truth is seen in a right leaning article entitled "Rachel was Wrong". The premise of the article was that the entire argument put forth by Rachel Carson's book *"Silent Spring"* was wrong. Yet the support put forth by the author to support her argument is seriously lacking. Statements without supportive facts is not science. Too much of what is passed as science today is merely opinion. In fact, the mantra of medicine is "evidence-based medicine". But what we really have is "marketing-based medicine". It is not the scientific evidence that is propelling the practice of providers, it is marketing and it's associated dollars.

Science has become politicized. As I stated above, politics has hijacked science to cloud truth for ideological purposes. Science should be used to generate thought and discussion. Instead, Science is being utilized to control thought and to control discussion.

Below are some of the political opinion statements masquerading as scientific fact from the above referenced article:

1) "pollution–including residue from pesticides–only accounts for 2 percent of all cancer"

The problem with this argument is everything. How in the world can one scientifically show that "only" 2 percent of all cancer are related to pesticides and other pollutants?! No data or reference is proposed to back up this claim by the author. Cancer is a multifactorial process involving epigenetics (disease as the result of a mix of genetics and environment), of which, environmental pollutants are just a fraction. We are all genetically predisposed to "X" disease or problem and it is environmental exposures/triggers that push us over the edge to disease.

2) "Most incidences of cancer stem from tobacco use or dietary choices"

This is an interesting point, as the "2 percent" referenced in point 1 typically comes from our dietary choices. The food that we eat, the water that we drink and bathe in, and the air that we breathe are all laced with varying levels of toxins. One cannot say that only 2 percent of cancers are caused by environmental toxins and then completely ignore their link with our food supply. The logic here is flawed; truth clouded by politics.

3) "humans aren't exposed to levels that are unsafe"

Says who? The CDC has recently said that no amount of exposure to lead in children is safe. A 2012 study found that "non-toxic" levels of 1 ppm (part per million) of glyphosate (component of Roundup) decreased Testosterone levels by 35%! In fact, Testicular cell damage occurs within 1 hour. And this is damage that is the result of an exposure considered non-toxic [452]!

The problem with toxins is they don't exist in a vacuum. If someone is exposed to lead; there are typically many other toxins they are dealing with at the same time. Nothing exists in a vacuum—toxins included. It would be inaccurate to claim that the Arsenic exposure from chicken provides an acute toxic dosage. However, Arsenic is found in water, timber, and the food supply (in the

---

452  Clair E et al. A glyphosate-based herbicide induces necrosis and apoptosis in mature rat testicular cells in vitro, and testosterone decrease at lower levels. Toxicol in Vitro. Mar 2012;26(2):269-79.

form of pesticides and insecticides). The point is, toxins are every-where. This volume of toxins strains our bodies detoxification system and lowers our effective threshold of toxicity. Glyphosate at low doses (36 ppm) will deplete the cell of its most important detoxifying molecule–glutathione [453]. And then consider how the government accepts and justifies mercury leakage from a new fluorescent lamp (CFL), and even mercury injected directly in to the bodies of developing children through thermerosol (known-ing children's brains are not fully developed until age 2)) and it becomes clear how fixed political ideology can lead to flawed sci-entific logic.

But back to the main point of this chapter–environmental impact on hormone receptors.

What is the relationship between environmental toxins and hor-mone receptors?

This relationship begins very, very early. In fact, before we are born. The perfect example is highlighted from a study published by UCSF in 2011 [454]. This study looked for 163 environmental toxins in 268 pregnant women. What they found was shocking. There were tox-ins present in all 268 pregnant mothers, some with as many as 43 separate toxins! And many of these toxic chemicals had not been commercially available for 30+ years. Think about that.

While folic acid is universally accepted as important in women desiring pregnancy and in early pregnancy, does that mean toxins like DDT, lead, and mercury are Ok in "safe" dosages. What is safe? Who defines safe? Arsenic is the most potent toxin

---

453   de Liz Oliveira Cavalli VL et al. Roundup disrupted male reproductive func-tions by triggering calcium-mediated cell death in rat testis and sertoli cells. Free Radic Biol Med. Jun 29 2013:pii:S0891-5849(13)00326-2.

454   Woodruff TJ, Zota AR, Schwartz JM. Environmental chemicals in pregnant women in the United States: NHANES 2003-2004. Environ Health Perspect. Jun 2011;119(6):878-885.

known to man. Is Arsenic safe in small dosages? I wouldn't place any bets on that with my family and I don't know anyone that would.

How do these toxins disrupt function? Most of these toxins in question are xenoestrogens. Xenoestrogens are natural or synthetic chemicals that have very weak estrogenic activity[455]. Xenoestrogens are 1,000 fold weaker than the most potent Estrogen[456]. They bind to the same ER alpha and ER beta discussed in the previous chapter and effect the cell's internal signaling. Xenoestrogens can also interfere via non-genomic pathways[457]. These xenoestrogens are above and beyond the estrogen made by the body thus increasing the overall effective estrogen level in the body. So, they act through the normal genomic and non-genomic pathways increasing the effective estrogen signal.

The perfect example of what can happen when exposure occurs during pregnancy is with diethylstillbestrol (DES). This was a synthetic estrogen used from 1940 to 1971 for the prevention of miscarriage and preterm labor. DES exposure resulted in significant female reproductive abnormalities (and in some cases, cancer)[458]. In males, DES exposure has been found to increase urogenital

---

455 Witorsch RJ. Endocrine disruptors: can biological effects and environmental risks be predicted? Regul Toxicol Pharmacol. Aug 2002;36(1):118-30.

456 Bouskine A et al. Low doses of Bisphenol A promote human seminoma cell proliferation by activating PK and PKG via a membrane G-protein-coupled estrogen. Environ Health Perspect. July 2009;117(7):1053-1058.

457 Nadal Angel et al. Nongenomic actions of estrogens and xenoestrogens by binding at a plasma membrane receptor unrelated to estrogen receptor alpha and estrogen receptor beta. PNAS. Oct 10 2000;97(21):11603-11608.

458 Herbst AL, Ulfelder H, Poskanzer DC. Adenocarcinoma of the vagina. Association of maternal stillbestrol therapy with tumor appearance in young women. N Engl J Med. 1971;284:878-881.

abnormalities [459] [460] [461] (to include epididymal cysts, undescended testes, smaller testes, and hypospadias). This was a very potent synthetic estrogen with powerful results.

Why DES? This book is about men? Correct, but DES exposure has been shown to have effects on males as well. Effects even before birth. The problem with DES in men, is that it changes the predominate estrogen receptor status from ER beta to ER alpha before birth. The feminizing effects of DES in men occurs through the ER alpha receptor [462] [463]. Again, this transformation occurs prior to birth with exposure to DES. Baby boys born during the DES years, had their response to estrogen altered prior to birth.

The perfect example of another xenoestrogen is bisphenol A (BPA). Bisphenol A is a xenoestrogen commonly found in plastics and is one of the more recognized xenoestrogens.

BPA, as a xenoestrogen, is a very weak estrogen receptor stimulator [464]. Many discount the impact of BPA due to its weak estrogenic activity. As weak as BPA is, it is ubiquitous in the environment. A prolonged exposure of a low potency toxin is just as dangerous as

459  Ross RK et al. Effect of in-utero exposure to diethylstilbestrol on age at onset of puberty and on postpubertal hormone levels in boys. Can Med Assoc J. May 15 1983;128(10:1197-8.

460  Kalfa N et al. Prevalence of hypospadias in grandsons of women exposed to diethylstilbestrol during pregnancy: a multigenerational national cohort study. Ferti Steril. Jun 30 2011;95(8):2574-7.

461  Klip H et al. Hypospadias in sons of women exposed to diethylstilbestrol in utero: a cohort study. Lancet. Mar 30 2002;359(9312):1102-7.

462  Couse JF, Korach KS. Estrogen receptor-alpha mediates the detrimental effects of neonatal diethylstillbestrol (DES) exposure in the murine reproductive tract. Toxicology. Dec 1 2004;205(1-2):55-63.

463  Walker VR, Jefferson WN, Couse JF, Korach KS. Estrogen receptor-alpha mediates diethylstilbestrol-induced feminization of the seminal vesicle in male mice. Environ Health Perspect. Apr 2012;120(4):560-5.

464  Timms BG et al. Estrogenic chemicals in plastic and oral contraceptives disrupt development of the fetal mouse prostate and urethra. Proceedings of the National Academy of Sciences. 2005.

a short exposure of a high potency toxin. One could argue that it is perhaps more dangerous due to it's indolent, gradual accumulation and effect.

The negative effects of BPA don't end there. What the body does with BPA is worse than the BPA itself. Scientists are discovering that the metabolites of BPA are equally prevalent and maybe even more toxic. One such metabolite, 4-methyl-2,4-bis(4-hydroxyphenyl) pent-1-ene or MBP for short, is found to have 1,000 times the estrogenic activity of BPA alone [465]. MBP makes up for the weak estrogenic activity of BPA. These potent estrogenic effects are occurring at very low levels of BPA exposure in people today. Most alarming, these levels are found in our children and are changing our children's response to hormones (estrogen receptors) before they are even born [466].

Xenoestrogen exposure starts very early. Bisphenol A has been shown to effect hormone receptor change at exposure levels between 1 picogram per million to 1 nanogram per million, and levels exceeding this have been found in pregnant mothers and their unborn children [467] [468] [469]. Bisphenol A has been shown to increase the estrogen and testosterone receptor expression in the

---

465  Okuda, T, Takiguchi M, Yoshihara S. In vivo estrogenic potential of 4-methyl-2,4-bis(4-hydroxyphenyl)pent-1-ene, an active metabolite of bisphenol A, in uterus of ovariectomized rats. Toxicol Lett. 2010;197:7-11.

466  Schonfelder G, Flick B, Malsness C, Paul M, Chahoud I. In Utero Exposure to low doses of Bisphenol A lead to Long-term deleterious effects in the Vagina. Neoplasia. March 2002;4(2):98-102.

467  Welshons WV, Nagel SC, vom Saal FS. Large Effects from small exposures. III. Endocrine mechanisms mediating effects of Bisphenol A at levels of human exposure. Endocrinology. June 1 2006;147(6):s56-s69.

468  Takahaski O, Oishi S. Disposition of orally administreed 2,2-Bis(4-hydroxyphenyl) propane (Bisphenol A) in pregnant rats and the placental transfer to fetuses. Environmental Health Perspectives. 2000;108:931-935.

469  Ikezuk Y et al. Determination of bisphenol A concentrations in human biological fluids reveals significant early prenatal exposure. Human Reproduction. 2002;17:2839-2841.

prostate prior to birth [470]. Additionally, bisphenol A shifts the estrogen receptors from a ER beta dominance to ER alpha dominance by increasing the encoding of ER alpha [471] [472]. This shift to ER alpha dominance favors inflammation and growth. All this in blood concentrations commonly found in humans.

So what does all this mean? With regards to Bisphenol A, exposure is changing the way we respond to hormones even before we are born. Bisphenol-A has been shown to increase estrogen receptor transcription (production at the DNA level) at very low levels of BPA (1 nM) in the prostate that is commonly found in blood today. Add in that the estrogen receptor production appears to be more of the alpha form [473] [474] [475], and we have a potential problem. The ER beta to ER alpha dominance change, discussed earlier, is not a good one physiologically. In review, ER alpha provides a more inflammatory and pro-growth interpretative signal from the estrogen message. In contrast, ER beta provides a more anti-inflammatory and anti-growth signal from the estrogen message. Second, the effects referenced above are found at levels that are far below that found

---

470  Richter CA et al. Estradiol and Bisphenol A stimulate androgen receptor and estrogen receptor gene expression in fetal mouse prostate mesenchyme cells. Environ Health Perspect. June 2007;115(6):902-908.

471  Monje L, Varayoud J, Luque EH, Ramos JG. Neonatal exposure to bisphenol A modifies the abundance of estrogen receptor alpha transcripts with alternative 5-untranslated regions in the femal rat preoptic area. J Endocrinol. July 1 2007;194:201-212.

472  Takao T et al. Exposure to the environmental estrogen bisphenol A differentially modulated estrogen receptor-alpha and beta immunoreactivity and mRNA in male mouse testis. Life Sci. Jan 24 2004;72(10):1159-69.

473  Richter CA et al. Estradiol and Bisphenol A stimulate androgen receptor and estrogen receptor gene expression in fetal mouse mesenchyme cells. Environ Health Perspect. Jun 2007;115(6):902-8.

474  Rajapakse N, Silva E, Kortenkamp A. Combining xenoestrogens at levels below individual no-observed-effect concentrations dramatically enhances steroid hormone action. Environ Health Perspect. 2002;110(9):917-921.

475  Welshons WV, Nagel SC, vom Saal FS. Large effects from small exposures. III. Endocrine mechanisms mediating effects of bisphenol A at levels of human exposure. Endocrinology. 2006;147(6 Suppl):S56-69.

in humans. These levels have been shown to contribute to abnormal male and female development. Additionally, BPA has been shown to contribute to adult sexual dysfunction, cognitive decline, immune dysfunction, and weight gain [476]. These negative effects of BPA have been found in both animal and human studies. [70].

If only the negative effect of xenoestrogens ended at the weak estrogenic activity and increased ER alpha production. We also know that bisphenol-A acts as an androgen receptor antagonist. Simply stated, bisphenol-A blocks the androgen receptor. Bisphenol-A disrupts the interaction between the androgens (DHEA, androstenedione, Testosterone, and DHT) with the androgen receptor [477] [478]. So, we have a commonly prevalent xenoestrogen, bisphenol-A, providing numerous effects (increased estrogen load, change in estrogen receptor expression, and blockade of the androgen receptor) that results in low Testosterone or low Testosterone signaling. Also know that bisphenol-A is only one of the many xenoestrogens that we are exposed to on a daily basis.

Just a sampling of these xenoestrogens include [479]:


- 4-Methylbenzyliden camphor (4-MBC) in sunscreen
- Butylated hydroxyanisole/BHA in food preservatives
- Atrazine in weedkiller
- Dieldrin in insecticides
- DDT in insecticides (yes this was banned many years ago)
- p,p'-DDE, a metabolite of DDT
- Endosulfan in insecticides

476   Richter CA. In Vivo Effects of Bisphenol A in Laboratory Rodent Studies. Reprod Toxicol. 2007;24(2):199-224.

477   Lee HJ, Chattopadhyay S, Gong EY, Ahn RS, Lee K. Antiandrogenic effects of bisphenol A and nonylphenol on the function of androgen receptor. Toxicol Sci. Sep 2003;75(1):40-6.

478   Curtis LR. Organophosphate antagonism of the androgen receptor. Toxicol Sci. 2001;60(1):1-2.

479   Melissa. "A List of Xenoestrogens." N.p., 20 Oct. Web.

- Erythrsine/FDC in red color dye
- Heptachlor in insecticide
- Lindane in insecticide
- Methyoxychlor in insecticide
- Nonylphenol and derivatives in surfactants, detergents, emulsifiers, and pesticides
- Parabens in lotions
- Phenosulfothiazine in red dye
- Phthalates in plastics
- DEHP in PVC
- Chlordecone in insecticide
- Fenitrothion, an organophosphate found in insecticides

There are many new xenoestrogens discovered almost every day. Though some of these xenoestrogenic sources have nothing to do with nutrition, many are common components of the farming industry and thus show up on/in our food products. Eventually, they contribute to the increase estrogenic load and contribute to low Testosterone. A recent tragedy highlights the danger of these xenoestrogens. In July of 2013, 21 school children, from the ages of 8 to 11, died after eating poisoned school lunches. Test results from the children revealed toxic levels of an organophosphate commonly found in insecticides. Organophosphates can be classified as a xenoestrogen. As you can see, xenoestrogens are not just endocrine disruptors, but are potentially very toxic–even deadly as in this tragic case.

The Environmental Working Group publishes an online list of the most toxic foods. Many of these toxins as you see above, are xenoestrogens masquerading as pesticides, insecticides and the like.

These toxins don't exist in a vacuum, don't exist alone and rarely are these toxins at "toxic" levels. In fact, levels below what is called "no observed effect" are shown to increase the effective hormone load [480]. Translation: very low levels of environmental toxins increase the internal hormone levels. This was referenced above with bisphenol A.

To say that the environment is not playing a role in our health is either ignorance, denial, or merely playing politics. The environmental impact on our health, has nothing to do with politics, but everything to do with truth. We need to remove our ideological blinders and analyze the scientific data as such.

It is one thing to be exposed to endocrine disrupting chemicals like bishphenol A and phthalates as an adult when full development has occurred. It is quite another to be exposed during the most critical developmental periods–in utero (in uterus embryologically). It is one thing to be exposed to just ONE environmental chemical toxin. It is all together a different thing to be exposed to hundreds, perhaps thousands of environmental toxins on a daily basis. This large volume of exposure in fact reduces the toxic threshold of the individual toxins. Additionally, negative effects have been found at levels far below the accepted toxic threshold levels for many of these environmental toxins [481].

Back to bisphenol A as our example. Bisphenol A is still in the environment and exposure is on going. Bisphenol A is a very weak estrogen [482] [483], no doubt, but the exposure is ubiquitous. A lot of

---

480  Rajapakse N, Silva E, Kortenkamp A. Combining Xenoestrogens at levels below individual no-observed-effect concentrations dramatically enhances steroid hormone action. Environ Health Perspect. Aug 2012;110:917-921.

481  Welshons WV, Nagel SC, Thayer KA, Judy BM, vom Saal FS. Low-dose bioactiviy of xenoestrogens in animals: fetal exposure to low doses of methoxychlor and other xenoestrogens increases adult prostate size in mice. Toxic Ind Health. 1999;15:12-25.

482  Tong W, Perkins R, Xing L, Welsh WJ, Sheehan DM. QSAR models for binding of estrogenic compounds to estrogen receptor alpha and beta subtypes. Endocrinology. 1997;138:4022-4025.

483  Kuiper GG, Carlsson B, Grandien K, Enmark E, Gagglbad J, Nilsson S, Gustafsson JA. Comparison of the ligand binding specificity and transcript tissue distribution of estrogen receptors alpha and beta. Endocrinology. 1997;138:863-870.

the research on endocrine disrupting chemicals (EDCs) has been on young ladies with precocious puberty (early development). It used to be that precocious puberty was defined as early sexual development at ages 10 and 11. Now it is 8 and 9 years of age. The question is, are we progressing in our development? Are we evolving into a higher species? Of course not. Our environment is effecting our development. Here in lies the example of bisphenol A (BPA) [484]. Bisphenol A has been shown to play a role in precocious puberty in young girls at even low exposure. Bisphenol A has been shown to be an estrogen receptor agonist [485] and in some cases an estrogen receptor antagonist [486]. Stated plainly, bisphenol A can act to stimulate estrogen receptors or bisphenol A can act to block estrogen receptors, depending on which receptor is involved [487]. Confused? That is because the effects of bisphenol A on receptors are not completely known, but we do know they interact with and alter the receptors.

But, what about the male counterpart?

Bisphenol A has been shown to have a wide spectrum of effects in boys and men today. Xenoestrogens have been shown to be endocrine disruptors at the level of the hypothalamus, pituitary, and the testes in pubertal development in young boys (see Figure 1) [488]. Estrogens and other xenoextrogens, like BPA, have been shown to decrease the expression of androgen receptors in the male prostate at high

484 Howdeshell KL, Hotchkiss AK, Thayer KA, Vandenbergh JG, vom Saal FS. Exposure to bisphenol A advances puberty. Nature. 1999;401:763-764.

485 Delfosse V et al. Structural and mechanistic insights into bisphenols action provide guidelines for risk assessment adn discovery of bisphenol A substitutes. PNAS. Sep 11 2012;109(37):14930-5.

486 Kurosawa T et al. The activity of bisphenol A depends on both estrogen receptor subtype and the cell type. Endocr J. Aug 2002;49(4):465-71.

487 Hiroi H, Tsutsumi O, Momoeda M, Takai Y, Osuga Y, Taketani Y. Differential interactions of bisphenol A and 17beta-estradiol with estrogen receptor alpha (ER alpha) and ERbeta. Endocr J. Dec 1999;46(6):773-8.

488 Zawatski W, Lee MM. Male pubertal development: are endocrine-disrupting compounds shifting the norms? J Endocrinol. Aug 1 2013;218:R1-R12.

doses [489] [490]. In contrast, bisphenol A has been shown to increase the expression of estrogen receptor alpha and increase the expression of androgen receptors in the prostate, with in utero exposure to bisphenol A [491]. This was found to occur at low levels, normally found in human serum. This effect is in a dose-dependent manner. Meaning, the higher the exposure: the greater the effect. Effects did occur at very low doses, at levels consistently in human blood.

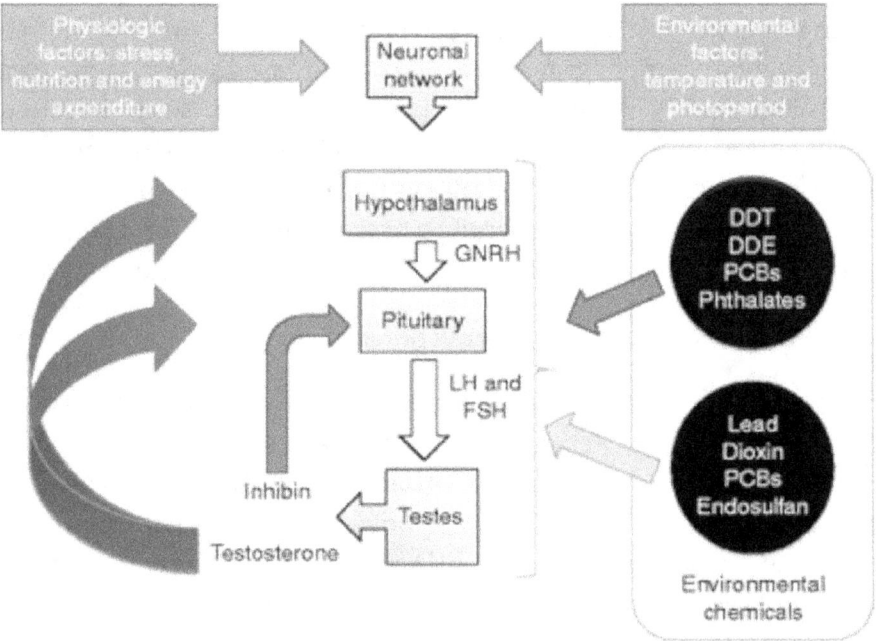

*(Figure 1 Endocrine disruptors effect on hormone production)* [39]

489  Prins GS, Birch L. The developmental pattern of androgen receptor expression in rat prostate lobes is altered after neonatal exposure to estrogen. Endocrinology. 1995;136:1303-1314.

490  vom Saal FS et al. Prostate enlargement in mice due to fetal exposure to low doses of estradiol or diethylstillbestrol and opposite effects at high doses. Proc Natl Acad Sci USA. 1997;94:2056-2061.

491  Richter CA, Taylor JA, Ruhlen RL, Welshons WV, vom Saal FS. Estradiol and Bisphenol A stimulate androgen receptor and estrogen receptor gene expression in Fetal mouse prostate mesenchyme cells. Environ Health Perspect. June 2007;115(6):902-908.

More alarming, is that xenoestrogen exposure is effecting males prior to birth. Bisphenol A has consistently been found to be present in fetal umbilical cord blood [492] [493] . A recent study found Bisphenol A and 2 of its metabolites (BPA glucuronide and BPA sulfate) in 100% of pregnancies evaluated through umbilical cord blood sampling [494]. Bisphenol A has been shown to increase androgen receptor and estrogen receptor alpha transcription with levels typical found in fetal exposure [495] [496]. This was shown to occur at levels of 1 picomole to 1 nanomole [497]. The point is: really small levels of bisphenol A effect change. Large levels on the order of Estradiol are not necessary to effect a change. This was confirmed by Taylor et al, who showed that low dose xenoestrogen exposure during fetal development does increase prostate growth and disease through increased estrogen receptor alpha expression [498]. Add in the decrease in ER beta expression (result of low

492  Chou Wei-Chun et al. Biomonitoring of bisphenol A concentrations in maternal and umbilical cord blood in regard to birth outcomes and adipokine expression: a birth cohort study in Taiwan. Environmental Health. 2011;10:94.

493  Fenichel P et al. Unconjugated bisphenol A cord blood levels in boys with descended or undescended testes. Hum Reprod. Apr 2012;27(4):983-90.

494  Gerona RR et al. BPA, BPA glucuronide, and BPA sulfate in mid-gestation umbilical cord serum in northern California cohort. Environ Sci Technol. Aug 13 2013. Epub ahead of print.

495  Schonfelder G, Wittfoht W, Hopp H, Talsness CE, Paul M, Chahoud I. Paren bisphenol A accumulation in human maternal-fetal-placental unit. Eviron Health Perspect. 2002;110:A703-A707.

496  Welshons WV, Nagel SC, Thayer KA, Judy BM, vom Saal FS. Low-dose bioactivity of xenoestrogens in animals: fetal exposure to low doses of methoxychlor and other xenoestrogens increases adult prostate size in mice. Toxicol Ind Health. 1999;15:12-25.

497  Welshons WV, Nagel SC, vom Saal FS. Large effects from small expsoures. III. Endocrine mechanims mediating effects of bisphenol A at levels of human exposure. Endocrinology. Jun 2006;147(6 suppl):S56-69.

498  Taylor JA, Richter CA, Ruhlen RL, vom Saal FS. Estrogen environmental chemicals and drugs: Mechanisms for effects on the developing male urogenital system. J Steroid Biochem Mol Biol. Oct 2011;127(1-2):83-95.

Testosterone) in the prostate [499] and the environment for a pro-inflammatory/pro-growth prostate is set. The effect is not just confined to the prostate. Estrogen receptor alpha and beta have been shown to increase in the pituitary [500] and the hypo-thalamus [501] as a result of bisphenol A exposure also.

All the negative press on bisphenol A has forced manufacturers to find replacements for bisphenol A. Unfortunately, the replacements, such as bisphenol S, are equally toxic [502].

All the above negative effects are just with one xenoestrogen. The point here is not to focus purely on bisphenol A, but to point out the environmental impact on the hormone signaling of our children's hormones even before birth. Throw into the mix the large volume of other xenoestrogens (remember the large exposure found in the UCSF study), add in endogenous estrogen production from aromatase activity, and you can see the potential problems in men. As Richter CA et al correctly concluded: "...serum estradiol may underestimate estrogen levels in prostate tissue because cells in the developing prostate express aromatase, which metabolized testosterone to estradiol and because estrogen receptor agonists, including xenoestrogens, exhibit additive effects in combination". It is not just a potential problem—it is a reality. It is likely worse than the current picture presents.

---

499  Hess-Wilson JK, Ho SM, Knudsen KE. Unique bisphenol A transcriptome in prostate cancer: novel effects on ER beta expression that correspond to androgen receptor mutation status. Environ Health Perspect. Nov 2007;115(11):1646-1653.

500  Khurana S, Ranmal S, Ben-Jonathan N. Exposure of newborn male and femal rats to environmental estrogens: delayed and sustained hyperprolactinemia and alter-ations in estrogen receptor expression. Endocrinology. Dec 2000;141(12):4512-7.

501  Monje L, Varayoud J, Luque EH, Ramos JG. Neonatal exposure to bisphenol A modi-fies the abundance of estrogen receptor alpha transcripts with alternatives 5-untrans-lated regions in the femal rat preoptic area. J Endocrinol. Jul 1 2007;194:201-212.

502  Vinas R, Watson CS. Bisphenol S disrupts estradiol-induced nongenomic signal-ing in a rat pituitary cell line: effects on cell functions. Environ Health Perspec. Jan 2013;121:352-358.

And all that is just dealing with estrogen receptors. Bisphenol A has been shown to suppress thyroid hormone receptors [503] [504], has been suggested to block progesterone receptors [505], has been shown to stimulate glucocorticoid receptors [506] [507], and has been shown to increase androgen receptors [508] as well. The point is xenoextrogens, like bisphenol A, have a wide spectrum of effects on hormone signaling.

The environment is changing how our bodies respond to hormones before we are born. Our genetics are not changing. That would take thousands of years. But the expression of our genetics are changing–this can happen in a generation.

We are almost left without a chance. How the signal is being interpreted by the receptors is being altered before the signal ever has a chance to relay its message. Remember: estrogen receptor alpha promotes an inflammatory and pro-growth signal. Xenoestrogen exposure increases ER alpha production. Add in, that low testosterone shifts ER beta to ER alpha dominance.

---

503  Sheng ZG, Tang Y, Liu YX, Yuan Y, Zhao BQ, Chao XJ, Zhu BZ. Low concentrations of bisphenol a suppress thyroid hormone receptor transcription through a nongenomic mechanism. Toxicol Appl Pharmacol. Feb 15 2012;259(1):133-42.

504  Iwamuro S, Yamada M, Kato M, Kikuyama S. Effects of bisphenol A on thyroid hormone-dependent up-regulation of thyroid hormone receptor and down-regulation of retinoid X receptor gamma in Xenopus tail culture. Life Sci. Nov 2 2006;79(23):2165-71.

505  Aldad TS, Rahmani N, Leranth C, Taylor HS. Bisphenol-A alters endometrial progesterone receptor expression in the nonhuman primate. Fertility and Sterility. July 2011;96(1):175-179.

506  Prasanth GK, Divya LM, Sadasivan C. Bisphenol-A can bind to human glucocorticoid receptor as an agonist: an in slico study. Journal of Applied Toxicology. 2009;30(8):769-774.

507  Sargis RM et al. Environmental endocrine disruptors promote adipogenesis in the 3T3-L1 cell line through glucocorticoid receptor activation. Obesity. 2010;18(7):1283-1288.

508  Wehterill YB, Petre CE, Monk KR, Puga A, Knudsen KE. The xenoestrogen bisphenol A induces inappropriate andrgoen receptor activation and mitogenesis in prostatic adenocarcinoma cells. Mol Cancer Ther. May 2002;1:515.

Then throw in the obesity problem and the resultant increased estrogen production through aromatase activity and you can see how men are dealing with a high estrogen problem and resultant low T. All result in a pro-inflammatory, pro-growth signal which is a set up for dysfunction and disease. And, it begins at conception.

# CHAPTER 11

# DETOXIFICATION

"For the first time in the history of the world, every human being is now subjected to contact with dangerous chemicals, from the moment of conception until death. In the less than three decades of their use, the synthetic pesticides have been so thoroughly distributed throughout the animate and inanimate world that they occur virtually everywhere."

Sounds like a quote you may have heard on the local news lately. But, it actually is from Rachel Carson's 1962 book *Silent Spring*.

Detoxification seems to be a buzz word these days. Just google detoxification and you will find everything from water detoxification to colon cleanses.

So, what is Detoxification?

Detoxification is defined as the chemical changes of a xenobiotic, a phytochemical or an endogenous (made by our own body) compound that renders it less toxic and ready to be excreted. Simply, detoxification is the means by which the body protects us from things that we take in from our environment or that which our own body makes. The body converts the toxic compound to a safer, more stable form for excretion to then be eliminated from the body.

Toxins in and Toxins out, right. Well, that is if everything is working as designed. There are many organs that detoxify. The skin (through sweating), kidneys (through...well guess)...every cell must detoxify. Even the gut is involved in detoxification. But the liver is probably the most important detox organ. The liver detoxification mechanism involves 2 main steps–Phase I and Phase II detoxification.

We are what we eat, drink, breath, and touch. But did you ever think that we are what we don't eliminate? Without elimination of the toxic chemicals we take in and produce every day, our bodies swim in a sludge pool of toxins. Nice visual, huh? This Increased toxic load on the body leads to inflammation. Inflammation will lead to disease and this will be covered in the last chapter on inflammation.

So, who needs detoxification?

Who needs detoxification and how would one know if they need detoxification? Look and listen to your body. This is something that women do well and something, that guys, we do not. The intuition of women has to be a God given gift. The body is going to tell you if it is in trouble or imbalanced. Whether through physical signs or symptoms, our bodies will let us know what is going on. Signs and Symptoms can be the bodies way of saying it is suffering from toxic build up. Symptoms are the way the body tries to get our attention that something is wrong.

A warning is meant to be heeded. A warning allows for early detection and will allow time for correction. In contrast, when a warning is ignored, destruction ensues.

What might be some warning signs? A few common signs and symptoms of toxin build up are:

- Headaches
- Muscle aches and pains
- Fatigue
- Asthma
- Allergies
- Skin disorders
- Chronic infections
- Altered mood
- Altered cognition
- Weight gain
- Altered stress tolerance
- Altered libido
- Infertility

Where do all these toxins come from? Toxins are ubiquitous. They are both exogenous and endogenous. The sources can range from toxins like heavy metals, pesticides, and insecticides, to merely taking to many prescriptions medications. For example, adverse reactions to prescription drugs have been ranked as the 4th to 6th leading cause of death in the US according to the Journal of American Medical Association [509]. This amounts to 100,000 deaths annually. A recent report from the Mayo Clinic found that 70% of Americans are on at least 1 prescription medication, 50% are on at least 2 prescription medications, and 20% are on at least 5 prescription medications[510]. Some perspective is always good. The 100,000 deaths is more than double those killed in car accidents annually. The

---

509  Lazarou J et al. Incidence of adverse drug reaction in hospitalized patients. JAMA. 1988;279(15):1200-1205.
510  Zhong W et al. Age and sex patterns of drug prescribing in a defined American population. Mayo Clinic Proceedings. July 2013;88(7):697-707.

cause, in part, is an overloaded pathway in Phase I detoxification. The specific phase I pathway involved is the CYP3A4. This phase I pathway (CYP3A4) is responsible for the detoxification of over 50% of all drugs. No wonder the people taking 5,6, and 7 prescription medications don't feel good. Their liver is crying for help! The costs associated with this pharmaceutical log-jam have been estimated at up to $4 billion. With the rising costs of health care, treating causes and decreasing prescription drugs would be a great way to prevent complications and lower costs. It would be a great way to improve detoxification. Looks like a good place to start.

The most dangerous sources of toxins are environmental–such as organochlorine pesticides, heavy metals, industrial chemicals, and unintended chemical byproducts. Most widespread production of these chemicals began 80 years ago. Our environment may have been highjacked by politics, but it is not a political issue. Recently the EPA estimated that 4 billion pounds of chemicals were released into the grounds natural water sources in 2000. The average American eats, unknowingly I might ad, 124 pounds of additives per year. And most people think America's problem are too many carbohy-drates. Over 2.5 billion pounds of pesticides are used on crop lands, forests, lawns, and fields. We surely live in a toxic world [511].

Our toxin load is the result of many sources. Here are some great ways to decrease your daily toxin exposure:

- Avoid processed foods
- Avoid trans and saturated Fats
- Avoid tap water; use filtered water
- Avoid excess caffeine
- Avoid excess alcohol

---

[511] "The Importance of Detoxification". Informational Brochure. (Advanced Nutrition Publications, Inc., 2002).

- NO tobacco
- Limit chronic medicine if possible
- regular exercise
- avoid liver dysfunction
- avoid kidney problems
- avoid intestinal dysfunction
- avoid occupational exposure
- avoid living near industrial plants
- avoid above the ground power lines

Obviously, some of the suggestions are easier to do than others–like avoiding occupational exposure and living near industrial plants. So, the better question is not who needs detoxification, but who does not need detoxification? Everyone can benefit from a periodic detoxification program. But, be very careful. Detoxification, if not properly managed, can make one feel worse. In fact, some detoxification program are counterproductive; these detoxification programs can themselves be the source of intermediate toxins due to increased phase I stimulation but inadequate phase II stimulation. Some of the toxic intermediates are more toxic than the initial toxic compound that needed detoxification to begin with.

How does one Detoxify?

Let's get down to the nuts and bolts of detoxification. We will use the liver as our reference example. The process of detoxification shows us how to detoxify. The proof is in the pudding as they say.

There are two parts to liver detoxification: Phase I and Phase II. Likened to Thing 1 and Thing II from Dr. Seuss. Phase 1 detoxification involves the cytochrome P450 system. The name comes from that fact that this system absorbs light at 450 nanometers. Phase I detoxification involves oxidation, reduction, and hydrolysis. Simply put, Phase I makes the parent compound (the toxin) more polar. Phase I detoxification is always active and is very redundant. What do I mean by redundant–there are many members of the CYP450 family, but there are over 200,000 substrates that use them. So, many different chemicals or substrates will use the same CYP450 enzyme. Remember the example about the CYP3A4 pathway? A great picture of the redundancy is seen at the Indiana University's school of medicine, division of clinical pharmacology at http://medicine.iupui.edu/flockhart/table.htm. This nice diagram reveals the commonly used CYP450 enzymatic pathways and the drugs used by these respective pathways. This diagram reveals the built in redundancy of the CYP pathways. This diagram should really put to rest the statement that detoxification is just a word used by "alternative" or "natural" doctors and has no intrinsic value other than detoxification from drugs and toxins. As if these pathways are only active when drugs such as heroin, alcohol, and cocaine need to be eliminated. If that is the case, then the Clinical Pharmacology division of Indiana University has either fabricated or wasted our time with this diagram. Of course, neither of those are true. These biochemical pathways of detoxification are active every second of every day! The idea that because we don't fully understand something, does not make that "something" invalid. Medicine is reeking with this concept problem.

But, it doesn't stop there. Phase I detoxification requires many cofactors:

- Niacin
- Magnesium
- Copper
- Zinc
- Vitamin C
- Vitamins B2, B3, B6, B12
- Folic acid
- Flavonoids

Vitamins are extremely important. Without them our bodies don't work well. A recent study on vitamins and cancer in 14,641 male physicians, found an 8% decrease in cancer in those regularly taking vitamins [512]. One more tidbit on vitamins. Did you know that many causes of vitamin deficiencies today are the prescription medications we take? A double whammy! The prescription medications we take to fix problems, simply cause deficiencies that can create more problems. We are ever chasing our tails.

Phase II [513] detoxification leads to further modification of the products of Phase I detoxification through conjugation. Essentially, large water-soluble molecules are added to the toxins through:

- Glutathione conjugation
- Amino acid conjugation
- Methylation
- Sulfation
- Acetylation
- Glucoronidation

Phase II detoxification is a very amino acid dependent process. If the diet of an individual is deficient in amino acids, it would be obvious to see how this could effect detoxification. Any detoxification program that has not evaluated these pathways and their intermediates will be woefully inadequate and potentially very dangerous. After phase II modification, the body is able to eliminate the inactivated toxins via the bowels and/or bladder.

In summary, Phase I and Phase II enzymes are the power houses that detoxify our bodies of our daily toxin load. They are very

512   Gaziano JM et al. Multivitamins in the prevention of cancer in men: the physicians health study II randomized controlled trial. JAMA. Nov 14 2012;308(18):1871-1880.
513   Liska DJ. The Detoxification Enzyme Systems. Altern Med Rev. 1998;3(3):187-198.

dependent on vitamins, minerals, amino acids, and energy. The many prescriptions we take lead to major drug interactions and vitamin depletions that interfere with our bodies ability to detoxify. Thus, if one is malnourished (typical American diet of fast food) and lacks key vitamins and nutrients, then our bodies cannot adequately detoxify. If we can't detoxify, we become inflamed, if we become inflamed, we develop disease. It can be that simple.

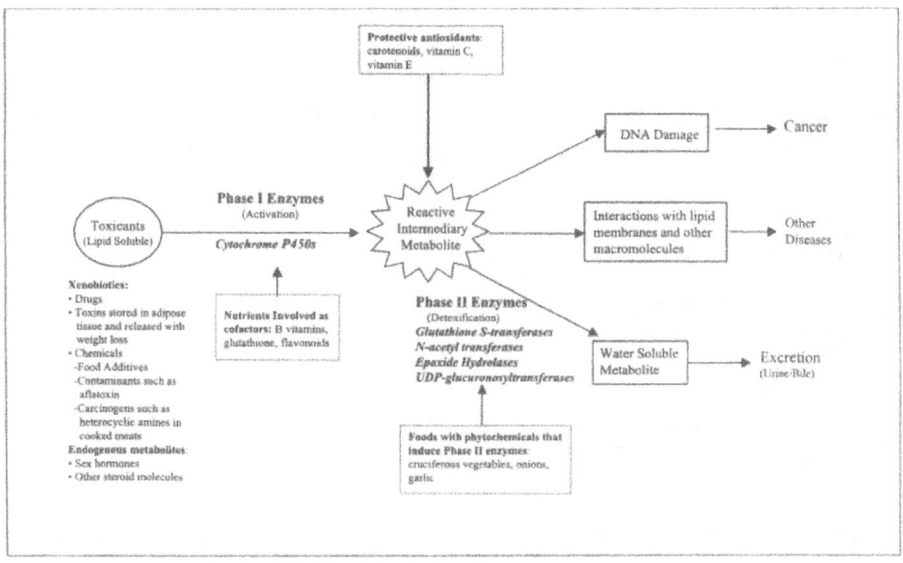

*(Figure 1 Detoxification)* [514]

Example?

Linear thinking would imply that Phase I and Phase II work together (i.e. when phase I is activated, then phase II is simultaneously activated). That is just not the case. Phase I pathways can be stimulated when phase II pathways are not, and vic versa. This itself can produce very toxic intermediates that are more dangerous to the body than the toxins it began with. The perfect example here is the drug

514  Patterson RE, Eaton DL, Potter JD. The genetic revolution: Change and challenge for the Dietetics profession. Journal of the American Dietetic Association. Nov 1999;99(11):1412-1420.

trileptal. Trileptal is an anticonvulsant commonly used in depression that induces the CYP3A4 enzyme. If the phase II pathways are not up the the challenge, so to speak, then you are left with a lot of toxic by-products due to upregulation in Phase I activity without Phase II support. And individuals that take these drugs are usually in no condition to handle any increase in toxic load.

The body has a way to handle these toxic intermediates– Glutathione. Glutathione is about the most important detoxification molecule in the body. The body uses glutathione to protect against the toxic by-products of detoxification. This is the bodies natural process for protecting against liver damage [515] from tylenol overdose [516] and chemotherapy toxicity [517]. The reduced form (H+ added) of glutathione is the active form. Once used, the body needs to make more glutathione or recycle the inactive glutathione. To recycle glutathione, the body uses vitamins like vitamin C [518], vitamin E [519], selenium [520], and zinc [521]. This is one of the reasons why

515  Dentico P et al. Glutathione in the treatment of chronic fatty liver diseases. Recenti Prog Med. Jul-Aug 1995;86(7-8):290-3.

516  Smith SW, Howland MA, Hoffman RS, Nelson LS. Acetaminophen overdose with altered acetaminophen pharacokinetics and hepatotoxicity association with premature cessation of intravenous N-acetylcysteine therapy. Ann Pharnacother. Sept 2008;42(9):1333-1339.

517  Smyth JF et al. Glutathione reduces the toxicity and improves quality of life of women diagnosed with ovarian cancer treated with cisplatin: results of a double-blind, randomised trial. Ann Oncol. 1997;8(6):569-573.

518  Carr AC, Frei B. Toward a new recommended dietary allowance for vitamin C based on antioxidant and health effects in humans. Am J Clin Nutr. Jun 1999;69(6):1086-1107.

519  Jain SK, McVie R, Smith T. Vitamin E supplementation restores glutathione and malondialdehyde to normal concentrations in erythrocytes of type 1 diabetic children. Diabetes Care. Sept 2000;23(9):1389-1394.

520  Venardos K, Harrison G, Headrick J, Perkins A. Effects of dietary selenium on glutathione peroxidase and thioredoxin reductase activity and recovery from cardiac ischemia-reperfusion. Journal of Trace Elements in Medicine and Biology. Sept 14 2004;18(1):81-88.

521  Cortese MM, Suschek CV, Wetzel W, Kroncke KD, Kolb-Bachofen V. Zinc protects endothelial cells from hydorgenperoxide via Nrf2-dependent stimulation of glutathione biosynthesis. Free Radical Biology and Medicine. June 15 2008;44(12):2002-2012.

vitamins C and E are so beneficial to the body and why I am such a proponent of vitamin C.

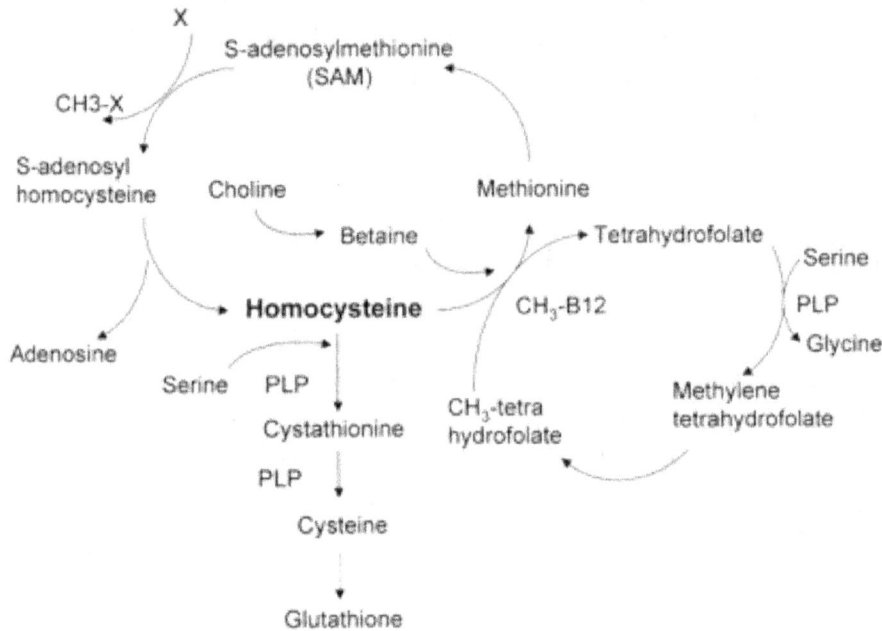

*(Figure 2 Inter-relation of trans-sulfuration and trans-methylation pathways)* [522]

The body can also make more glutathione through the trans-sulfuration pathway [523]. The trans-sulfuration pathway is a deviation away from the methylation pathway (see figure above). The center spoke, so to speak, is homocysteine. Homocysteine can be a biomarker used to assess cardiovascular (CVD) risk. Older studies revealed associated increased CVD risk with an elevated homocysteine [524] [525].

522   Cravo ML, Camilo ME. Hyperhomocysteinemia in chronic alcoholism: relations to folic acid and vitamins b6 and b12 status. Nutrition. April 2000;16(4):296-302.

523   McBean GJ. The transsulfuration pathway: a source of cysteine for glutathione in astrocytes. Amino Acids. Jan 2012;42(1):199-205.

524   Wald DS, Law M, Morris JK. Homocysteine and cardiovascular disease: evidence on causality from a meta-analysis. BMJ. Nov 23 2002;325(7374):1202.

525   Refsum H, Ueland PM, Nygard O, Vollset SE Homocysteine and cardiovascular disease. Annual Review of Medicine. Feb 1998;49:31-62.

Likely, homocysteine does not "cause" CVD [526], but is the result of the cause, which is high detoxification demand and thus a decrease in methylation and a rise in homocysteine to feed the glutathione pathway for detoxification. This results from the bodies ability to manipulate biochemical pathways. If the body requires more glutathione due to increased demand, then the body will down regulate methionine synthase (the enzyme that converts homocysteine to methionine) to feed precursors to the glutathione production pathway. The mere presence of some toxins can themselves inhibit methionine synthase and result in an increase in homocysteine levels. This has been shown to be one of the pathway dysfunctions found in children with autism [527]. Lead, and to a stronger degree Mercury, can inhibit the enzyme methionine synthase at very, very low levels (1 nM) [528]. It doesn't take a lot of toxin exposure to increase glutathione production through the trans-sulfuration pathway and slow the methylation pathway through inhibition of methionine synthase.

One of the precursor to glutathione is cysteine. Cysteine can be provided through N-acetyl-cysteine, also known as NAC. This is the treatment of choice for liver toxicity due to tylenol overdosage [529]. It is no surprise that NAC promotes glutathione production to aid detoxification of the liver in similar situations and protect against liver damage [530].

526  Clarke R. Homocysteine and coronary heart disease: Meta-analysis of MTHFR case-control studies, avoiding publication bias. PLoS Med. Feb 2012;9(2):e1001177.

527  James SJ et al. Metabolic biomarkers of increased oxidative stress and impaired methylation capacity in children with autism. Am J Clin Nutr. Dec 2004;80(6):1611-1617.

528  Stajich GV, Lopez GP, Harry SW, Sexson WR. Iatrogenic exposure to mercury after hepatitis B vaccination in preterm infants. J Pediatr. May 2000;136(5):679-81.

529  Smith SW, Howland MA, Hoffman RS, Nelson LS. Acetaminophen Overdose with Altered acetaminophen pharmacokinetics and hepatotoxicity associated wth premature cessation of intravenous N-acetylcysteine therapy. Ann Pharmacother. Sept 2008;42(9):1333-1339.

530  Dentico P et al. Glutathione in the treatment of chronic fatty liver diseases. Recenti Prog Med. Jul-Aug 1995;86(7):290-3.

This is the reason why I am opposed to general detox programs in a bottle. I have seen many detoxification programs result in side effects due to inadequate support in particular pathways. Detoxification in a bottle does not provide customized support to match the specific individual's needs. Do these individuals have Phase I problems, Phase II problems, glutathione problems or a combination thereof? Are these pathways compromised due to exposure of toxins or are they compromised due to genetics? The purpose of detoxification is to aid the body in its elimination of toxins. Inadequate support can actually aid the toxin build up.

How about some solutions?

There are a few general supplements that do provide general detoxification support that I highly recommend.

NAC

N-actyl-cysteine (NAC) is the precursor to glutathione. I mentioned above that NAC is the treatment of choice for tylenol liver toxicity. It has been shown that tylenol induces CYP 450 (Phase I detoxification) pathway which results in an increase in the toxic intermediates previously discussed. This results in glutathione depletion [531]. Depletion of glutathione allows oxidative damage and hepatotoxicity. NAC protects the liver against this oxidative damage from the tylenol toxicity through increased glutathione production.

Glutathione is not readily bioavailable through oral administration and therefore intravenous therapy is the best choice to give glutathione. Glutathione is a great therapy IV and has been shown to aid Parkinson's disease [532], reduce toxicity of chemo-

---

531  James LP, Mayeux PR, Hinson JA. Acetaminophen-induced hepatotoxicity. DMD. Dec 2003; 31(12):1499-1506.

532  Sechi G et al. Reduced intravenous glutathione in the treatment of early parkinson's disease. Progress in Neuro-Psychopharmacology and Biological Psychiatry. Oct 1996;20(7): 1159-1170.

therapy [533], aid septic shock treatment [534], and protect against non-alcoholic fatty liver disease [18]. The only reliable effective method to increase glutathione via the oral route is with NAC. NAC is a great antioxidant in any oral regimen. N-acetyl-cysteine is best taken at 1,200 mg in two divided doses. That would be 600 mg twice daily. There are no known side effects of NAC orally at these dosages.

Sulforaphane

Many supplements have dual action. Sulforaphane is the perfect example. As further discussed in the chapter on inflammation, Sulforaphane is a powerful anti-inflammatory. However, sulforophane is a potent stimulator of Phase II detoxification as well [535]. Sulforphane is found in the well known cruciferous vegetables–so eat plenty of broccoli, brussel sprouts and the like to support phase II naturally. However, to get the therapeutic dosages describe in the scientific literature, one would have to eat more broccoli than many of us would care to eat in a day. Phase II inducers support the elimination of Phase I intermediates and aid in the clearance of the toxic intermediates. To achieve higher dosing than that available through dietary intake, sulforaphane must be dosed orally through supplement form. A good oral dosage of sulforaphane is 200 mg taken in divided dosing. Sulforophane is very safe with no side effects. But of course, remember what your mom said and eat more broccoli.

---

533  Cascinu S, Cordella L, Del Ferro E, Fronzoni M, Catalano G. Neuroprotective effect of reduced glutathione on cisplatin-based chemotherapy in advanced gastric cancer: a randomized double-blind placebo-controlled trial. JCO. Jan 1996;13(1):26-32.

534  Ortolani O et al. The effect of glutathione and N-acetylcysteine on lipoperoxidative damage in patients with early septic shock. Am J Respir Crit Care Med. Jun 1 2000;161(6):1907-1911.

535  Morimitsu Y et al. A sulforaphane analogue that potently activates the Nrf2-dependent detoxification pathway. The Journal of Biological Chemistry. Feb 1 2002;277:3456-3463.

## DIM

Diindolylmethane (DIM) is a metabolite of another commonly employed supplement indole-3-carbinol (I3C). DIM is also derived from cruciferous vegetables. DIM has been shown to slow cancer cell growth [536] [537]. Part of the benefit of DIM is through its induction of Phase II detoxification [538]. A good daily regimen of DIM is 300 mg taken in divided dosages. DIM is very safe and there are no known side effects of DIM at these dosages.

But of course, the best way to provide good detoxification support is through a balanced diet rich in cruciferous vegetables. Diets rich in cruciferous vegetables have been shown to reduce the incidence of prostate [539] [540], colorectal (sorry guys, women only) [541], lung (again women only) [542], and breast cancer [543]. These studies

536 Pappa G et al. Quantitiative combination effects between sulforaphane and 3,3'-diindolylmethane on proliferation of human colon cancer cells in vitro. Carcinogenesis. 2007; 28(7):1471-1477.

537 Chen I, McDougal A, Wang F, Safe S. Aryl hydrocarbon receptor-mediated anti-estrogenic and antitumorigenic activity of diindolylmethane. Carcinogenesis. 1998;19(9):1631-1639.

538 Nho CW. Jeffery E. Crambene, a bioactive nitril derived from glucosinolate hydrolysis, acts via the antioxidant response element to upregulate quinone reductase alone or synergistically with indole-3-carbinol. Toxicology and Applied Pharmacology. Jul 1 2004;198(1):40-48.

539 Kolonel LN et al. Vegetables, fruits, legumes and prostate cancer: a multethinic case-control study. Cancer Epidemiology, Biomarkers Prevention. 2000;9(8):795-804.

540 Jain MG, Hislop GT, Howe GR, Ghadirian P. Plant foods, antioxidants, and prostate cancer risk: findings from case-control studies in Canada. Nutrition and Cancer. 1999;34(2):173-184.

541 Voorrips LE et al. Vegetable and fruit consumption and risks of colon and rectal caner in a prospective cohort study: The Netherlands Cohort Study on Diet and Cancer. American Journal of Epidemiology. 2000;152(11):1081-1092.

542 Feskanich D et al. Prospective study of fruit and vegetable consumption and risk of lung cancer among men and women. Journal of the National Cancer Institute. 2000;92(22):1812-1823.

543 Terry P, Wolk A, Persson I, Magnusson C. Brassica vegetables and breast cancer risk. JAMA. 2001;285(23):2975-2977.

are not absolute. However, they show that cruciferous vegetables provide significant health benefits. It is interesting that cruciferous vegetables are primarily winter vegetables. They provide many health benefits at the same time some illnesses (i.e. flu and cold) are on the increase.

Cruciferous vegetables are the source of Diindolylmethane, indole-3-carbinol, and sulforophane mentioned above. In addition, they are a good source of vitamin E, vitamin A, vitamin K, folic acid and micronutrients. One would have to eat a WHOLE lot of veggies to get the benefit provided in the supplement listed dosing above. But, daily intake of cruciferous vegetables are a great basic start to any detox program and why not make detoxification a part of your daily diet. It is cheaper, easier, and tastes a lot better to just eat your detoxification support.

Below is a list of common cruciferous vegetables to add to your diet:

- Arugula
- Bok Choy
- Broccoli
- Brussels sprouts
- Cabbage
- Cauliflower
- Chinese cabbage
- Collard greens
- Daikon radish
- Horseradish
- Kale
- Kohlrabi
- Land cress
- Mustard greens
- Radish

- Rutabaga
- Shepherd's purse
- Turnip
- Watercress

Eat up, detoxify, and enjoy!

# CHAPTER 12

---

# INFLAMMATION

What is inflammation?

You are not alone if this question stumps you. Blank stares with visible question marks is the response I normally get. As discussed in previous chapters, inflammation actualy is a normal physiologic process. Inflammation is the product of the communication between the different parts of the immune system. In the short-term, inflammation protects and initiates the healing process. But in the long-term, when unchecked and with no off switch, chronic inflammation can be self-directed and cause serious damage—even death. A normal physiologic process designed to protect and heal, if dysfunctional, can be the cause of disease that ends life. Amazingly delicate balance.

Chronic Inflammation is a prerequisite for most chronic diseases of aging. Again, we are not talking about the acute inflammatory response, but the low-grade, chronic, unchecked inflammation that flies under the radar. The obvious examples here are auto-immune diseases. Autoimmune disease is simply the immune system attacking the body. Examples here include Hashimoto's thyroid disease, Lupus, Ankylosing Spondylitis, and Rheumatoid arthritis–but there are many more.

What if I told you Type II diabetes, hypertension, cardiovascular disease, obesity, and cancer have all been shown to be the result of chronic inflammation? In fact they have. The majority of this inflammation has been shown to originate from the gut. Specifically the gut bacteria. Shocked? Most are.

This inflammatory process has been coined "metabolic endotoxemia". Metabolic endotoxemia is when a high fat diet alters the gut bacterial balance. A high fat diet is also referred to as overnutrition and Dietary Induced Obesity (DIO). This altered gut bacterial balance results in increased intestinal permeability. This increased intestinal permeability results in increase blood lipopolysaccharide (LPS) levels resulting in increased inflammation. So simply stated: metabolic endotoxemia is dietary induced, gut altered, systemic inflammation that increases disease. Got it. Obesity is not just calories in and calories out! No linear thinking when it comes to the body's physiology. Metabolic endotoxemia (see figure 1 below) has been show to either initiate or play a significant role in insulin resistance [1], obesity, [544], diabetes [545], non-alcoholic fatty liver disease (NAFLD) [546], metabolic syndrome [547], and atherosclerosis [548]. One could say that metabolic syndrome is the doorway to disease. It can

---

544  Cani PD et al. Metabolic endotoxemia initiates obesity and insulin resistance. Diabetes. Jul 2007;56(7):1761-72.

545  Pussinen PJ et al. Endotoxemia is associated with an increased risk of incident Diabetes. Diabetes Care. Feb 2011;34(2):392-397.

546  Alisi A, Ceccarelli S, Panera N, Nobili V. Causative role of gut microbiota in non-alcoholic fatty liver disease pathogenesis. Front Cell Infect Microbiol. 2012;2:132.

547  Manco M. Endotoxin as a missed link among all the metabolic abnormalities in the metabolic syndrome. Atherosclerosis. 2009;206:36-;author reply 37.;author reply 37.

548  Wiesner P et al. Low doses of LPS and minimally oxidized LDL cooperatively activate macrophages via NF-KappaB and AP-1: possible mechanims for acceleration of atherosclerosis by subclinical endotoxemia. Circ Res. July 9 2010;107(1):56-65.

be said that inflammation arising from the gut plays a role in chronic diseases of aging. Unregulated inflammation equals disease.

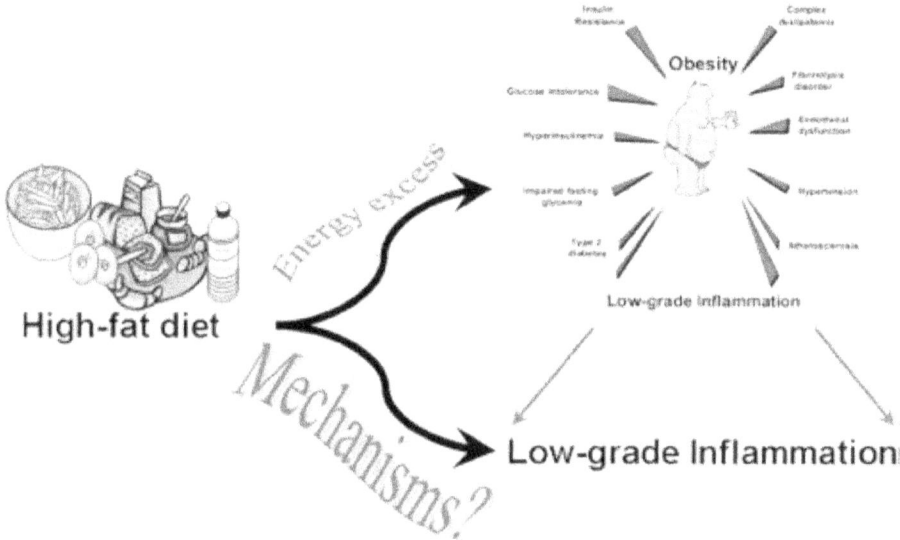

*(Figure 1 High-fat to obesity through metabolic endotoxemia)* [549]

Back to the basics. What is inflammation? I hear many clinicians traveling the country discussing inflammation like it is some kind of alter ego or something. Inflammation, like stress, is a biochemical process and needs to be taken seriously. Inflammation is how the immune system communicates. Inflammation is normal and then inflammation is not normal.

Make sense?

Inflammation in the short term is good. Let's take the example of a paper cut. Inflammation is responsible for protecting against secondary invasion of bacteria and starting the process of healing. The immune system signals and attracts cells, like macrophages,

---

549  Cani PD, Delzenne NM. The role of the gut microbiota in energy metabolism and metabolic disease. Current Pharmaceutical Design. 2009;14:1546-1558.

to the sight of injury to protect against foreign invasion and start the process of healing. Once these goals are accomplished, inflammation resolves. Contrast this with chronic inflammation–where the immune system chatter never turns off. This constant inflammatory response has consequences. And the consequence is collateral damage. It is this chronic inflammation that is linked with dysfunction and disease that is the subject of this chapter.

But first, a brief summary of the immune system. The immune system is divided into two essential parts: the innate immune system and the humoral immune system. Common active cells in the immune system are monocytes, macrophages, natural killer cells... The macrophages and the neutrophils constitute the innate immune system and the lymphocytes (B type and T type) constitute the humoral or adaptive immune system. These immune cells can have dual action in both the innate and humoral immune systems. For example, the innate immune system is involved in the first line of defense against many common pathogens. But, the innate immune system is also involved in the signaling to the humoral immune system to provide more specific, adaptive immune responses. Lets say for example, you are exposed to a bacteria through the gastrointestinal system. The macrophages would engulf the bacteria to destroy it, but at the same time would process that pathogen to then present to other cells to signal for more macrophages (innate) and antibody production (adaptive immunity). There is a primary role, but there is cross talk to ensure adequate protection.

The innate immune system is the first line of defense. The innate immune system is like the first wave of the army in a ground attack. Their mission is to hit the beach and gain a foothold. Fighting is close quarters and often hand to hand. The innate immune system is non-specific. The innate immune system is non-specialized and protective against a limited number of bacteria, viruses, and parasites.

Contrast this with the humoral immune system. The humoral immune system is often referred to as the acquired or adaptive immunity. The humoral immune system is like the artillery. They are not involved in hand to hand combat, but instead prosecute specific measures of attack against specific targets. The humoral immune system is highly specialized, adaptable, and is very active against the majority of the pathogens that we encounter. The humoral immunity is also delayed compared to the immediate action of the innate immunity–about 4-7 days. This is the antibody part of the immune system [550].

One can see that the innate and the humoral immune systems need to communicate. What is this communication? The language of the immune system are cytokines and chemokines. Cytokines are how the immune system communicates. Chemokines attract more immune cells to the sight of action. The mere presence of inflammation means your immune system is active and communicating and that is good. Look at the cardinal symptoms of inflammation: redness, pain, swelling, and heat. The mere presence of inflammation does not imply dysfunction. Again, inflammation in the presence of surgery is normal and needed to heal and repair, but chronic low-grade inflammation, such as that found in type II diabetes and obesity, is not.

The cytokines or chemical messengers of the immune system arise from cells called T helper cells. T helper cells are activated by the macrophages of the innate immune system discussed above. As in the innate and humoral immunity, there seem to be 2 primary divisions of the T helper cells. The T helper 1 (Th1) cells are primarily associated with innate immunity signaling. Th1 cells signal the cells of the innate immune system. T helper 1 cells secrete the cytokines Interleukin 2, Tumor Necrosis factor alpha, Interferon-gamma, and Interleukin-12. The Th1 cells are responsible for most of the

550  Janeway CA Jr, Travers P, Walport M et al. *Immunobiology: The Immune system in Health and Disease*. 5th Edition. New York: Garland Science; 2001.

traditional signs of inflammation discussed above. In contrast, the T helper 2 cells (Th2) are primarily concerned with the humoral or adaptive immunity. Th2 cells secrete interleukins 4, 5, 9, 10, and 13 to name a few. Th2 cells stimulate B cells to produce antibodies. T helper 2 cells are thus highly associated with allergic reactions [551].

The paradigm of the Th1 and Th2 system originated in the 1980s with Mosmann [552] [553]. New discoveries and knowledge occur all the time in medicine. The world of immunology (immune system) is no different. Since 1980, a third subset of T cells have been discovered. This subset is called T helper 17 (Th17). This subset of T cells is particularly inflammatory. T helper 17 cells are active against extremely pathogenic bacteria, active against pathogens that escape Th-1 defenses, and has been linked to autoimmune disease development [554] [555] [556] [557] [558]. T helper 17 cells, like Th1 and Th2, have their own set of inflammatory cytokines–IL17 type A -F, IL-21, and IL-22 [559].

551 Alberts B, Johnson A, Lewis J et al. Helper T cells and Lymphocyte activation. Molecular Biology of the Cell. 4th edition. New York: Garland Science; 2002.

552 Mosmann TR. T lymphocyte subsets, cytokines, and effector functions. Ann N Y Acad Sci 1992;664:89-92.

553 Mosmann TR, Cherwinski H, Bond MW, et al. Two types of murine helper T cell clone: I. Definition according to profiles of lymphokine activities and secreted proteins. J Immunol 1986;136:2348-2357.

554 Bettelli E, Korn T, Kuchroo VK. Th17: The third member of the effector T cell Trilogy. Curr Opin Immunol. Dec 2007;19(6):652-657.

555 Steinman L. A brief history of T(H)17, the first major revision in the T(H)1/T(H)2 hypothesis of T cell-mediated tissue damage. Nat Med. 2007;13:139–145.

556 Steinman L. A brief history of T(H)17, the first major revision in the T(H)1/T(H)2 hypothesis of T cell-mediated tissue damage. Nat Med. 2007;13:139–145.

557 Chen Y, Langrish CL, McKenzie B, Joyce-Shaikh B, Stumhofer JS, McClanahan T, Blumenschein W, Churakovsa T, Low J, Presta L, et al. Anti-IL-23 therapy inhibits multiple inflammatory pathways and ameliorates autoimmune encephalomyelitis. J Clin Invest. 2006;116:1317–1326.

558 Bettelli E, Carrier Y, Gao W, et al. Reciprocal developmental pathways for the generation of pathogenic effector TH17 and regulatory T cells. Nature 2006;441:235-238.

559 Nurieva R, O Yang X, Martinez G, Zhang Y, Athanasia D, Ma L, Schluns K, Tian Q, Watowich SS, Jetten M, et al. Essential autocrine regulation by IL-21 in the generation of inflammatory T cells. Nature. 2007.

Let's look at the example of metabolic endotoxemia again to further explain the effects of cytokines, inflammation, and disease. In the beginning, there is a high fat diet (HFD) or excess energy intake. This can also be referred to as Dietary induced obesity (DIO). The point here is a lot of us eat too many empty calories devoid of any nutritional value. The high fat diet results in an imbalance in the delicate gut bacterial population. The gut bacterial imbalance is referred to as dysbiosis. This imbalance in the gut bacterial population creates inflammation. The systemic effects of this inflammation is called endotoxemia and this has been shown to result in obesity and diabetes [560].

Let's go deeper. The high fat diet [2][561] is the cause of the imbalanced gut bacteria [7]. The result is an increase in lipopolysaccharide (LPS) levels. The LPS is a major component of the outer membrane of gram-negative bacteria that is the result of the increase in the gut gram negative to gram positive balance–also called dysbiosis. The resultant LPS has been shown to be the cause of inflammation [562] that is found in neuroinflammation and neurodegeneration [563][564][565], insulin resistance [566]

---

560  Cani PD et al. Changes in gut microbiota control metabolic endotoxemia-induced inflammation in high fat diet-induced obesity and diabetes in mice. Diabetes. 2008;57:1470-1481.

561  Ghanim H et al. Increase in plasma endotoxin concentrations and the expressio of Toll-like receptors and suppressor of cytokine signalin-3 in mononuclear cells after a high-fat, high-carbohydrate meal: implications for the insulin resistance. Diabetes Care. 2009. 32:2281-2287.

562  Martich GD, Boujoukos AJ, Suffredini AF. Response of man to endotoxin. Immunobiology. Apr 1993;187)3-5):403-16.

563  Qin L et al. Systemic LPS causes chronic neuroinflammation and progressive neurodegeneration. Glia. Apr 1 2007;55(5):453-62.

564  Lee DC et al. LPS-induced inflammation exacerbates phopho-tau pathology in rTg4510 mice. Journal of Neuroinflammation. 2010;7:56.

565  Lee JW et al. Neuro-inflammation induced by lipopolysaccharide causes cognitive impairment through enhancement of beta-amyloid generation. Journal of Neuorinflammation. 2008;5:37.

566  Arkan MC et al. IKK-beta links inflammation to obesity-induced insulin resistance. Nature Medicine. 2005;11:191-198.

[567], diabetes [568], abnormal cholesterol levels [569], and obesity [570]. All the result of the high fat diet. Poor nutrition found in a high fat diet [2] is the cause of the increase in gram-negative dysbiosis, which results in the increased LPS levels. The result is inflammation.

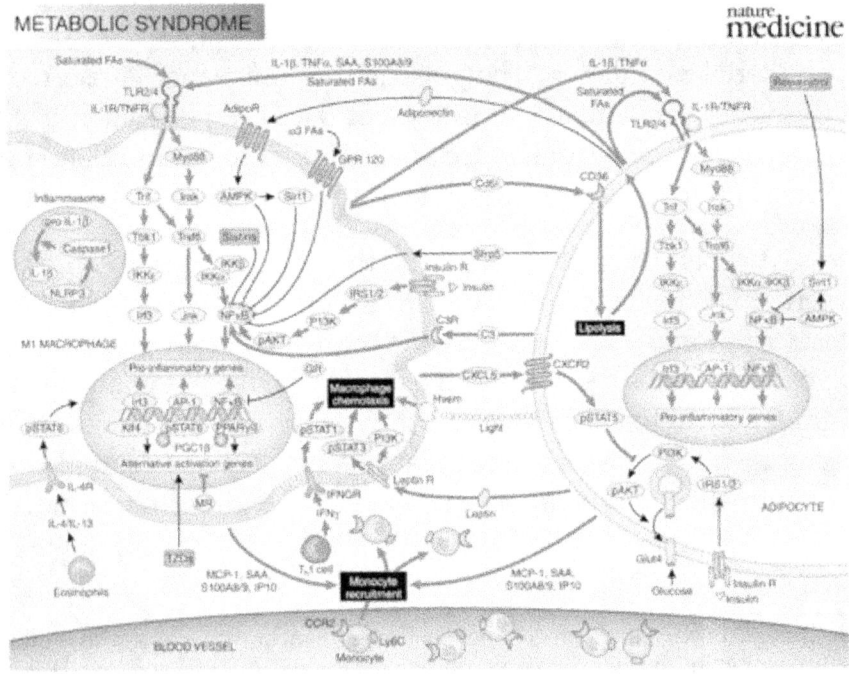

*(Figure 2 Biochemistry of Metabolic Syndrome)* [571]

567   Agwunobi AO et al. Insulin resistance and substrate utilization in human endo-toxemia. J of Clin Endocrinol Metab. June 6 2000;85(10):3770-3778.

568   Pussinen PJ, Havulinna AS, Lehto M, Sundvall J, Salomaa V. Endotoxemia is associated with an increased risk of incident diabetes. Diabetes Care 2011;34:392–397.

569   Lassenius MI et al. Bacterial endotoxin activity in human serum is associated with dyslipidemia, insulin resistance, obesity, and chronic inflammation. Diabetes Care. Aug 2011;34(8):1809-1815.

570   Kim KA et al. High fat diet-induced gut microbiota exacerbates inflammation and obesity in mice via the TLR4 signaling pathway. PLoS ONE. Oct 16 2012;7(10):e47713.

571   Nguyen KD, Chawla A. Metabolic Syndrome ePoster. Nature Medicine. http://www.nature.com/nm/poster/eposter_full.html.

The negative impact of a high fat diet is not just the empty calories. A high fat diet is itself a cause of inflammation directly. A high fat diet is indirectly a cause of inflammation through altered gut bacteria balance.

This is a paradigm shift–that the bacterial imbalance in the gut can be the cause of obesity. I have referenced the impact of gut bacterial balance and inflammation above. Two specific bacterial populations have been linked to inflammation and obesity–Bacteroidetes and Firmicutes. A decrease in the Bacteroidetes:Firmicutes (2 prominent bacteria in the gut) ratio has been shown to be associated with obesity and diabetes in animal studies. Animals with this balance have significant fat accumulation, metabolic dysfunction, and inflammation in the presence of a high fat diet. In contrast, animals without a low Bacteroidetes:Firmicutes ratio will stay lean, even in the presence of a high fat diet [572] [573] [574]. These same findings have been shown in humans as well [575]. In contrast, a 2011 study found no correlation with carbohydrate and fat intake. But a high fat diet was associated with a trend in Firmicutes increase and those with a high carbohydrate diet trended to an increase in both Firmicutes and Bacteroidetes. A significant association with Firmicutes and hsCRP (a marker of systemic inflammation) was found [576].

Remember, a high fat diet alters the gut bacterial balance. This altered gut bacterial balance in turn can favor a trend or absolute

---

572   Backhed F et al. The gut microbiota as an environmental factor that regulates fat storage. Proce Natl Acad Sci U S A. 2004;101(144):15718-15723.

573   Backhed F et al. Mechanism underlying the resistance to diet-induced obesity in germ-free mice. Proce Natl Acad Sci U S A. 2007;104(3):979-984.

574   Turnbaugh PJ et al. An obesity-associated gut microbiome with increased capacity for energy harvest. Nature. 2006;444(7122)1027-1031.

575   Ley RE et al. Microbial ecology: human gut microbes associated with obesity. Nature. 2006;444(7122):1022-1023.

576   Ismail NA et al. Frequency of Firmicutes and Bacteroidetes in gut microbiota in obese and normal weight Egyptian children and adults. Arch Med Sci. June 2011;7(3):501-507.

change in the energy extraction from food. Both result in an increase in systemic inflammation and metabolic dysfunction.

All these effects might be ok if they stayed confined to the gut. But, of course that is not the case. The increased LPS starts to effect the fat tissue. Remember, adipose tissue is biologically active. There are what are called adipose tissue macrophages (ATM). These ATMs are attracted to the growing adipose tissue. It has been estimated that 20-30 million macrophages accumulate for every 2.2 lbs of accumulated fat [577] [578]. Just think about that picture for a minute.

The increase in LPS levels increase the expression of Toll-like receptors (TLRs) on the the migrating macrophages [579] [580]. Through the increase in TLR-4 expression, both LPS and a high fat diet can increase intracellular inflammatory signaling through NF-kappaB activation [581]. The increased LPS additionally, causes a shift in the immune cells in the fat tissue. The immune cells, called macrophages here, shift from an anti-inflammatory signaling effect to one of a more pro-inflammatory effect. Have we seen this before? Yes we have–remember the estrogen receptors. Specifically, for you biochemistry detail junkies, there is a shift from M2 type macrophage to a M1 type macrophage in the fat tissue. The result is a shift from an anti-inflammatory, metabolically neutral fat tissue to an inflammatory, increased metabolic

---

577 O'Rourke RW et al. Depot-specific differences in inflammatory mediators and a role for NK cells and IFN-gamma in inflammation in human adipose tissue. Int J Obes (Lond). 2009;33(9):978-990.

578 Lumeng CN, Saltiel AR. Inflammatory links between obesity and metabolic disease. J Clin Invest. 2011;121(6):2111-2117.

579 Akira S, Takeda K, Kaisho T. Toll-like receptors: critical proteins linking innate and acquired immunity. Nat Immunol;2:675-680.

580 Tajima T et al. Lipopolysaccharide induces macrophage migration via prostaglandin D2 and prostaglandin E2. JPET. Aug 2008;326(2):493-501.

581 Tsukumo DM, Carvalho-Filho MA, Carvalheira JBC, et al. Loss-of-function mutation in Toll-like receptor 4 prevents diet-induced obesity and insulin resistance. Diabetes. 2007;56:1986–98.

dysfunctional fat tissue. This metabolically dysfunctional and pro-inflammatory fat tissue actually has a name based on its appearance. It is called a crown-like structure [582] [583].

The LPS interacts with the M1 macrophages of the crown-like structure. This interaction occurs at specific receptors called Toll-like receptors (remember, that the LPS increases the expression of the TLRs). Toll-like receptors (TLR) are expressed on the fat cell macrophages and are activated by the increased LPS. The activated TLR then transfers the signal to the nucleus of the macrophage to transcribe inflammation through NF-kappaB [584]. NF-kappaB is a nuclear transcription factor through which inflammation is transcribed. The result is a production of inflammatory cytokines– TNF-alpha, IL-6, IL-1B, IFN-gamma [585] [586] [587] [588] [589] [590] [591]. So, you might describe NF-kappaB as the key to turn on inflammation.

582  Altintas MM et al. Mast cells, macrophages, and crown-like structures distinguish subcutaneous from visceral fat in mice. J Lipid Res. Mar 2011;52(3):480-8.

583  Khan T et al. Metabolic dysregulation and adipose tissue fibrosis: role of collagen VI. Mol Cell Biol. Mar 2009;29(6):1575-1591.

584  Muzio M, Polentarutti N, Bosisio D, Manoj, Kumar PP, Mantovani A. Toll-like receptor family and signaling pathway. Biochem Soc Trans. 2000;28:563-566.

585  Applied Biosystems. User Bulletin #2: ABI Prism Sequence Detection System. 2001.

586  Collart MA, Baeurele P, Vassalli P. Regulation of tumor necrosis factor alpha transcription in macrophages: involvement of four kappa B-like motifs and of constitutive and inducible forms of NF-kappa B. Mol Cell Biol. 1990;10:1498-1506.

587  Feta A, D'Agostino R Jr, Tracy RP, Haffner SM. Elevated levels of acute-phase proteins and plasminogen activator inhibitor-1 predict the development of type 2 diabetes: the Insulin Resistance Atherosclerosis Study. Diabetes. 2002;51:1131-1137.

588  Kern PA, Ranganathan S, Li C, Wood L, Ranganathan G. Adipose tissue tumor necrosis factor and interleukin-6 expression inhuman obesity and insulin resistance. Am J Physiol Endocrinol Metab. 2001;280:E745-E751.

589  Libermann TA, Baltimore D. Activation of interleukine-6 gene expression through the NF-kappa B transcription factor. Mol Cell Biol. 1990;10:2327-2334.

590  Senn JJ, Klover PH, Nowak IA, Mooney RA. Interleukin-6 induces cellular insulin resistance in hepatocytes. Diabetes. 2002;51:3391-3399.

591  Uysal KT, Wiesbrock SM, Marino MW, Hotamisligil GS. Protection from obesity-induced insulin resistance in mice lacking TNF-alpha function. Nature. 1997;389:610-614.

These inflammatory cytokines (that originate from fat), also referred to as adipocytokines, contribute to major metabolic dysfunction. The innate immune system activity signaling is the disrupting signal that contributes to a lot of disease. For example, Tumor Necrosis Factor alpha (TNF-alpha) actually causes a disruption in the GLUT-4 receptor that leads to insulin resistance and type II diabetes [592] [593]. Additionally, these inflammatory cytokines cause a decrease in the pancreatic islet cells in the pancreas causing a precipitous drop in insulin production, through pancreatic islet cell death [594] [595]. The result is an increase in insulin requiring diabetes [596]. These studies provide a direct biochemical link between inflammation and insulin dysfunction that can result in Diabetes.

So, what was the point of reviewing the biochemistry behind metabolic endotoxemia? An intellectual exercise perhaps? To reveal the complexity of the body and disease generation? To ooh and aah you? No. The review of the biochemistry behind metabolic endotoxemia is simply to reveal how inflammation plays a key role, if not an absolute step, in the genesis of disease. Next, to show what inflammation is and how inflammation has an impact on normal physiology resulting in dysfunction and disease. Additionally, to show the dynamic interaction of the body. The balance or imbalance in the body. And finally, to show that the current dogma of linear thinking in medicine and disease is obsolete.

---

592  Stephens JM, Lee J, Pilch PF. Tumor necrosis factor-alpha-induced insulin resistance in 3Ts-L1 adipocytes is accompanied by a loss of insulin receptor substrate-1 and GLUT4 expression without a loss of insulin receptor-mediated signal transduction. J Biol Chem. Jan 10 1997;272(2):971-6.

593  Lorenzo M et al. Insulin resistance induced by tumor necrosis factor-alpha in myocytes and borwn adipocytes. J Anim Scie. Apr 2008;86(14 Suppl):E94-104.

594  Cnop M et al. Mechanisms of Pancreatic Beta cell death in Type I and Type II diabetes. Diabetes. Dec 2005;54(2):S97-S107.

595  Eizirik DL, Mandrup-Poulsen T. A choice of death: the signal transduction of immune-mediated Beta-cell apoptosis. Diabetologia. 2001;44:2115-2133.

596  Wang C, Guan Y, Yang J. Cytokines in the progression of pancreatic Beta-Cell dysfunction. International Journal of Endocrinology. 2010;

Inflammation is amazing!

Inflammation is helpful.

Inflammation is dangerous.

Inflammation effect hormones.

Hormones effect inflammation.

Poor diets high bad fats are only one path to inflammation. Now let's look at Estradiol. Estradiol is an Estrogen. Sorry to bust your bubble guys, but we men make Estrogen (review the chapter on hormones). Some of us make a lot of Estrogen. And no, you can't predict based on the clothes that men wear.

This should come as no surprise to anyone. One of the primary causes of low Testosterone in men is a high Estrogen level–thus the purpose of this book. I propose that low Testosterone is the effect and not the cause. Estradiol and Estrone (estrogens) will feed-back to the hypothalamus and pituitary and shut off Testosterone production. This disruption even occurs at the site of the testicle. Estrogens can be endogenous (what your body makes) or exogenous (from the environment also known as xenoestrogens). In addition, Estrogens promote inflammation as we will discuss below. This inflammation influences the environment in which Testosterone exists and thus influences the signal of Testosterone and DHT [597].

There are several reasons that testosterone levels in American men are at an all time low–stress, weight, endogenous estrogens and xenoestrogens. See chapter 4 for a review on the causes of low Testosterone in men.

---

597 Osterlund KL, Handa RJ, Gonzales RJ. Dihydrotestosterone alters cyclooxygen-ase-2 levels in human coronary artery smooth muscle cells. American Journal of Physiology. Endocrinology and Metabolism 2010;298:E838-E845.

What is the problem with estrogen in men? Is it the the driving force behind the metrosexual male? NO. One of the problems with estrogen in men, is that it drives inflammation.

But how?

First, high endogenous estrogen levels in men come through high aromatase activity. Aromatase is the enzyme that converts Androstenedione and Testosterone into Estrone and Estradiol respectively [598]. Aromatase is present in many different tissues, but in men aromatase activity is highly concentrated in that mid-life bulge around the mid-section.

Hormones are not just about numbers, but balance and metabolism as well. Unfortunately, aromatase activity in men increases with age, stress, weight, and inflammation. None of us are going to get away from aging (right there with death and taxes). And who do you know that has NO stress? In fact, it is estimated that 90% of doctor visits are stress-related. Additionally, as we age, we gain weight and have more inflammation. That "age-related" tire around the mid-section is more than just unsightly–it is a hormone, inflammatory producing organ. Adipose tissue is biologically active. And remember the metabolic endotoxemia discussed above? This is inflammation arising from the GI system, causing obesity, which turns right around and produces inflammation. Vicious cycle! And guess what is concentrated in fat? That is right–aromatase activity. Aromatase activity in men accounts for 80% of estrogen production [599].

Second, high estrogen in men can be the result of massive over-dosage of testosterone. What? You mean one can dose too high on

---

598   Santen RJ, Brodie H, Simpson ER, Siiteri PK, Brodie A. History of Aromatase: Saga of an Important Biological Mediator and Therapeutic Target. Endocrine Reviews June 1 2009;30(4):343-375.

599   Vermeulen A, Kaufman JM, Goemaere S, van Pottelberg I. Estradiol in elderly men. Aging Male. Jun 2002;5(2):98-102.

testosterone? Yes, and most men prescribed Testosterone today are overdosed. Doping is not something that just happens in athletics. Doping is common place today in hormone replacement therapies. In my practice we have seen many men that have had to donate blood due to excess production of hemoglobin and hematocrit because of testosterone overdosage. This polycythemia, as it is called, is dangerous and unnecessary [600]. As a 20-22 year old, we men only would produce 5-10 mg daily [601]. And do you remember what you were like in your early 20s? Ahhh...the glory days. But, did you have to donate blood monthly due to your peak testosterone production? Of course–the answer is no. So, if you didn't have to donate blood with your peak testosterone production in your 20s, you shouldn't have to donate with testosterone therapy in your 40s and beyond either. The starting dosage for one of the most prescribed androgen gels commercially available today is 40 mg daily. If we didn't need 40 mg of testosterone in our early 20s, then we don't need it beyond our 30s. More is not always better. If 80% of a man's Estrogen production occurs from aromatase activity and aromatase activity increases as we age, are we not just throwing fuel on the fire with these massive doses? We physicians forget our physiology. Sorry, more is not better–even if it is something your body needs.

Third, is the delivery method. Testosterone secretion follows a normal diurnal rhythm. Testosterone levels are known to be greatest in early morning and lowest in the evening. Today, it is very common to get weekly Testosterone shots or Testosterone pellets placed every 3-4 months. What is physiologic about that? The answer is of course–nothing. Studies don't show that Testosterone peaks occur weekly or every 3 months. The problem with these methods are the

---

600 Hajjar RR, Kaiser FE, Morley JE. Outcomes of Long-term Testosterone replacement in older hypogonadal males: A retrospective analysis. The Journal of Clinical Endocrinology % Metabolism. Nov 1 1997;82(11):3793-3796.

601 Korenman SG, Wilson H, Lipsett MB. Testosterone production rates in normal adults. Journal of Clinical Investigation. 1963;42(11):1753-1760.

supra-physiologic peaks they produce. These delivery methods take Testosterone to places they were never intended to be. Our creator sure didn't intend for us to get Testosterone that way. I don't remember Adam getting his Testosterone injection or pellets in the Garden of Eden. A good friend of mine reminded me that Adam didn't get Testosterone in a cream either. But, at least transdermal Testosterone closely mimics the bodies production and release of Testosterone.

The effects of Testosterone to Estrogen conversion in men and women are different. That should come as no surprise to anyone. The practice of medicine should follow scientific literature, not opinion or marketing. In men, high aromatase activity and conversion of Testosterone to Estrogen has been linked to elevated C-reactive protein (CRP) [602] [603] [41], fibrinogen [604] [605], and IL-6 [606]. Are these inflammatory markers important? C-reactive protein is one of the best indicators of future cardiovascular disease/events (heart attacks and strokes), and is associated with metabolic syndrome [607] [608] [609]. Yes, it is even more predictive than cholesterol

602  Burney BO et al. Low testosterone levels and increased inflammatory markers in patients with cancer and relationship with cachexia. J Clin Endocrinol Metab. May 2012;97(5):E700-9.

603  Kapoor D, Clarke S, Stanworth R, Channer KS, Jones TH. The effect of testosterone replacement therapy on adipocytokines and C-reactive protein in hypogonadal men with type 2 diabetes. Eur J Endocrinol. May 1 2007;156:595-602.

604  Malkin CJ, Pugh PJ, Jones TH, Channer KS. Testosterone for secondary prevention in men with ischaemic heart disease? QJM. 2003;96(7):521-529.

605  Barud W et al. Relation between markers of inflammation and estradiol in older men. Med Sci Monit. Dec 2010;16(12):CR593-7.

606  Maggio M et al. Estradiol and inflammatory markers in older men. J Clin Endocrinol Metab. 2009;94:518-522.

607  Toss H, Lindahl B, Siegbahn A, Wallentin L. Prognostic influence of increased fibrinogen and C-reactive protein levels in unstable coronary artery disease. Circulation. 1997;96:4204-4210.

608  Ridker PM, Buring JE, Cook NR, Rifai N. C-reactive protein, the metabolic syndrome, and risk of incident cardiovascular events. Circulation. 2003;107:391-397.

609  Devaraj S, Singh U, Jialal I. Human C-reactive protein and the metabolic syndrome. Curr Opin Lipidol. Jun 2009;20(3):182-189.

levels [610]. Fibrinogen is another marker of inflammation that has been associated with cardiovascular disease and systemic inflammation. Interleukin-6 is an inflammatory cytokine (immune signal) that has been implicated in increased aromatase activity (conversion of Testosterone to Estrogen) and at the same time is the result of increased Testosterone to Estrogen activity.

Inflammation does not just end there. The adipocytokines IL-6 and TNF-alpha have been shown to disrupt the hypothalamic-pituitary axis. The adipocytokines, IL-6 and TNF-alpha, actually inhibit the release of the gonadotropins–leutinizing hormone (LH) and follicle stimulating hormone (FSH) from the pituitary. The result is a decrease in signal to the testicles to produce both Testosterone and sperm. This is also known as the hypogonadal-obesity-adipocytokine hypothesis [611] [612]. Meaning: low testosterone increases weight gain, which increases inflammation. Or is it, obesity increases inflammation that causes low T? But, it may be Inflammation causes low T, which causes weight gain. The point is, the low T, obesity, and systemic inflammation can become a vicious cycle.

If low Testosterone and increased Estrogen production in men increases inflammatory biomarkers like CRP, then Testosterone therapy should reduce these inflammatory biomarkers. That is in fact the case. A 2010 study in Clinical Endocrinology, found that Testosterone supplementation in men with metabolic syndrome reduced inflammatory biomarkers [613]. Testosterone has also been

---

610  Ridker PM, Rifai N, Rose Lynda, Buring JE, Cook NR. Comparison of C-reactive protein and low-density lipoprotein cholesterol levels in the prediction of first cardiovascular events. N Engl J Med. 2002;347:1557-1565.

611  Jones TH. Testosterone associations with erectile dysfunction, diabetes and the metabolic syndrome. 2007. Euro Urol Suppl;6:847-857.

612  Kelly DM, Jones TH. Testosterone: a metabolic hormone in health and disease. J Endocrinol. June 1 2013;217:R25-R45.

613  Kalinchenko SY et al. Effects of testosterone supplementation on markers of the metabolic syndrome and inflammation in hypogonadal men with the metabolic

shown to inhibit the production of IL-6, IL1-beta, CRP and TNF-alpha [614] [615] [616] [617].

So, all men should take testosterone? The answer is No. Remember the environmental influence of Testosterone on tissue. If the cause of low T is obesity and/or inflammation and we give Testosterone, then we are just throwing fuel on the fire.

The studies are not 100% conclusive. They never are. According to the scientific literature, it is clear that inflammation increases Testosterone to Estrogen conversion through increased aromatase activity. The increased Estrogen production is associated with increased inflammation in men. What a vicious cycle!

It does not end there. Leptin is another hormone that got a lot of attention back in the late 90's. Leptin is a hormone released from adipose tissue (remember that fat is biologically active) in response to the positive energy balance–to much stored fat. Normally, leptin induces LH release from the pituitary. However, in the overweight or obese individual, the pituitary become leptin resistant. This is very similar to insulin resistance. Back to a previously used analogy–when you ask your kids to clean their room the first time, your voice is low and calm. With each successive repeat of the

syndrome: the double-blinded placebo-controlled Moscow study. Clin Endo. Nov 2010;73(5):602-612.

614 Hatakeyama H et al. Testosterone inhibits tumor necrosis factor-alpha-induced vascular cell adhesion molecule-1 expression in human aortic endothelial cells. FEBS Letters. 2002;530:129-132.

615 Kelly DM, Jones TH. Testosterone: a vascular hormone in health and disease. J Endocrinol. June 1 2013;217:R47-R71.

616 Malkin et al. The effect of testosterone replacement on endogenous inflammatory cytokines and lipid profiles in hypogonadal men. Journal of Clinical Endocrinology and Metabolism. 2004;89:3313-3318.

617 Kalinchenko SY et al. Effects of testosterone supplementation on markers of the metabolic syndrome and inflammation in hypogonadal men with the metabolic syndrome: the double-blinded placebo-controlled Moscow Study. Clinical Endocrinology. 2010;73:602-612.

statement, "clean your room" the tone and volume of the statement gets louder and louder. This is exactly what is happening here. The fat knows that the pituitary is not listening (resistance) and so the fat starts to yell at the pituitary. Thus, inflammation results in the Leptin resistance at the level of the pituitary causing a rise in leptin levels [618].

It is at the level of the pituitary that Leptin normally stimulates Testosterone production through LH release in response to the increasing abdominal fat. However, in the Leptin resistant individual, this does not happen and the much needed increase in Testosterone production does not materialize. If it only ended there. The increase in the Leptin levels inhibit the LH stimulation of the leydig cells of the testes. The leydig cells are the cells that make Testosterone. Thus, inflammation results in Leptin resistance. The Leptin resistance results in an increase in Leptin levels. The result is a decrease in testosterone production at both the pituitary level and the testes level [619].

What is the big deal? No pun intended. The big deal is: insulin resistance, hypertension, prostatitis, cardiovascular disease, auto-immune disease, and cancer. Just too name a few.

I can hear the question now–the Testosterone a man needs can lead down the path of disease? If you give supra-physiologic levels, don't follow the levels, and don't monitor the balance and metabolism, it sure can. That is why I like to evaluate hormones first with saliva. As stated in a 2006 article, "plasma levels of Estradiol do not necessarily reflect tissue-level activity" [35]. Saliva has been shown to reveal the active hormone inside the cell at the site of action. Remember, the classical genomic receptors are inside the

---

618 Jones TH. Testosterone associations with erectile dysfunction, diabetes and the metabolic syndrome. European Urology Supplements. 2007;6:847-857.

619 Isidori AM. Leptin and androgens in male obesity: evidence for leptin contribution to reduce androgen levels. The Journal of Clinical Endocrinology Metabolism. Oct 1 1999;84(10):3673-3680.

cell. Then, one must follow hormones levels to ensure proper levels of hormones and proper balance of hormones. Finally, how the Estrogens are metabolized play an equally pivotal role in hormone effect and risk [620]. This is the only way to ensure that the Testosterone given to men is raising the Testosterone and DHT levels instead of being converted all to Estrogen. Hormone therapy is safe. However, hormone therapy must be properly evaluated, properly dosed, and properly followed.

Another very important hormone that can effect the immune system is Cortisol. Cortisol is the fight or flight hormone produced and released from the adrenal glands. Cortisol is essential for life. You can't live without it. Cortisol trumps all other hormones. When in survival mode, all other tasks (sex, bowels, sleep...) are not important. High cortisol in times of stress is one of the main causes of low testosterone. When stressed, sex can be difficult (though sex can be a great stress relief), sleep is difficult, and constipation is common.

Low Cortisol has been associated with increased inflammation [621], such as increased IL-6 cytokine production [622] [623]. Low cortisol has been associated with poor outcomes following strokes [624], burns,

---

620 Cutolo M. Estrogen metabolites: increasing evidence for their role in rheumatoid arthritis and Systemic Lupus Erythematosus. J of Rheumatol. Mar 2004;31(3):419-421.

621 Fries E, Hesse J, Hellhammer J, Hellhammer DH. A new view on hypocortisolism. Psychoneuroendocrinology. Nov 2005;30(10):1010-1016.

622 Remmelts HH et al. Biomarkers define the clinical response to dexamethasone in community-acquired pneumonia. J Infect. Jul 2012;65(1):25-31.

623 Rohleder N, Joksimovic L, Wolf JM, Kirschbaum C. Hypocortisolism and increased glucocorticoid sensitivity of proinflammatory cytokine production in Bosnian war refugees with posttraumatic stress disorder. Biological Psychiatry. Apr 2004;55(7):745-751.

624 Marklund N, Peltonen M, Nilsson TK, Olsson T. Low and high circulating cortisol levels predict mortality and cognitive dysfunction early after stroke. J Inter Med. Jul 2004;256(1):15-21.

and septicemia [625] [626]. The mechanism behind the poor outcome is thought to be inflammation. Hormones effect the immune system. Vice versa, the immune system effects hormones.

If inflammation is so instrumental in disease, then reducing inflammation should be a major part of any preventative or health wellness program. I am always amazed at how little attention is giving to inflammation. As it relates too inflammation, it all starts with what we eat. The previous chapter on nutrition addressed diet, but let's review nutrition as it relates too inflammation.

The old adage, "you are what you eat" couldn't ring more true. I don't like using the word "diet" as it has such a negative connotation in our culture. As the saying goes, "the only thing a diet does is help one to start to die". In my practice, I focus on healthy living to lose weight. One can lose weight in a healthy or in an unhealthy manner. But if one loses weight the right way, through life style changes focused on healthy living, then weight loss is a by product of improved physiologic function. Health is the result. In that sense, I view obesity and overweight as symptoms of poor health–no different than any other symptom that one may have as a result of poor health.

The process of inflammation reduction starts with eliminating inflammatory foods from your diet. There are a couple of ways to do this. First, eat a healthy, balanced diet. When I am on the road I am always amazed at the dietary choices people make. A diet coke and cookies for a diabetic on the airplane. A hotdog with chili for breakfast in the airport. All of these are real life examples and they were all obese. These individuals were making extremely poor dietary choices at the most important of times.

---

625   Aygen B, Inan M, Doganay M, Kelestimure F. Adrenal functions in patients with sepsis. Exp Clin Endocrinol Diabetes. 1997;105:182-6.

626   Cooper MS, Stewart PM. Corticosteroid insufficiency in acutely ill patients. N Engl J Med. 2003;348:727-34.

As I previously discussed, a high fat diet in the presence of an imbalanced gut bacteria population is a recipe for inflammation and fat production. But, the presence of macronutrient imbalance is also critical in inflammation. We have 3 macronutrients in our diet: amino acids, essential fatty acids, and carbohydrates. A "balanced diet" is referencing a balance of these macronutrients. Unfortunately, the SAD American diet is anything but balanced. The American diet is high in carbohydrates, especially refined or simple carbohydrates (think sugar) and high in fats. Some fats are good (omega-3). Some fats are bad (saturated and trans fats). The imbalance of these individual macronutrients is also a source of inflammation.

Breakfast, as they say, is the most important meal of the day. Studies have shown that eating a high quality breakfast, consisting of protein in the morning, increases the metabolic rate for the day. Conversely, skipping breakfast or a poor quality breakfast that is high in carbohydrates (especially simple sugars), decreases the metabolic rate for the day [627] [628]. Of course, this is effected by the health status of the individual. The point is balance. Look at the typical American breakfast: cereal, bagels, toast, donuts, bread–carbohydrates and sugars! According to the USDA in 1989, the annual dietary sugar intake of an adult 12-29 equated to 638 cans of soda, 135-200 lbs of refined sugar, 90 lbs of fat, 63 dozen donuts, 60 lbs of cake/cookies, 22 lbs of candy, and 15 lbs of chips/popcorn/pretzels. That is total. Hungry anyone? I think it would be safe to say that that number has probably gone a lot higher.

---

627  Astbury NM, Taylor MA, Macdonald IA. Breakfast consumption affects appetite, energy intake, and the metabolic and endocrine responses to foods consumed later in the day in male habitual breakfast eaters. J Nutr. Jul 2011;141(7):1381-9.

628  Marjan J van Erk, Blom WA, Ommen BV, Hendriks Henry FJ. High-protein and high-carbohydrate breakfasts differentially change the transcriptome of human blood cells. Am J Clin Nutr. Nov 2006;84(5):1233-1241.

It was Hippocrates that said, "let food be your medicine and medicine be your food". The more appropriate saying for Americans today is–let food be your poison and poison be your food.

Now, I don't want you to think I am the food police. I eat some foods high in fat and carbohydrates. But the appropriate term is "some", "few", and "limited". My metabolism is good. But my metabolism has not always been good. The metabolisms of some individuals are so dysfunctional that they cannot cheat once. When they cheat, their negative effects are exponentiated. When I cheat, my metabolism handles it. That is the effect of different states of health.

Back to the diet. The American Diet is very imbalanced. Whether it be a high carbohydrate, a high fat, or just a high intake of everything (remember dietary induced obesity), Americans diets are imbalanced. Simply restoring balance in the macronutrients will often result in weight loss, which will reduce inflammation. This is one of the reasons why amino acids and Omega-3s are often included in weight loss programs. The addition of the amino acids help to restore balance in addition too providing fuel for muscle growth. Muscle has a high capacity to burn fat. Embedded within muscle are mitochondria. Mitochondria are called the power houses of the cell because their job is to make energy. For those of you that had to live through the nightmare that was biochemistry, that is what glycolysis, the Kreb's cycle, and the Electron Transport Chain are all about.

The second way to reduce inflammation in your diet is to balance the fat intake. In addition too restoring dietary balance, omega-3's reduce inflammation [629], reduce sudden death [630], reduce

---

629   Kiecolt-Glaser JK et al. Omega-3 supplementation lowers inflammation in healthy middle-aged and older adults: A randomized controlled trial. Brain, Behavior, and Immunity. Aug 2012. 26(6):988-995.

630   Marchioli R et al. Early protection against sudden death by n-3 polyunsaturated fatty acids after myocardial infarction: time-course analysis of the results of

cardiovascular disease [631], and reduce triglyceride production. Triglycerides [632], whether in the blood or stored, are fat. But you must take in fat to lose fat. I know it seems counterintuitive, but the proper balance of fat intake is important. Just as the fats must be balanced with the other macronutrients, the types of fats must also be balanced, specifically omega-3's and the omega-6's need to be balanced. The intake of saturated fats, trans fats, and omega-6's, which are very pro-inflammatory, must be balanced by the anti-inflammatory omega-3's. Just look at the inuit eskimos. They eat a ton of fat and smoke like chimney stacks, yet their risk of cardiovascular disease is quite low [633]. Why? Their balance of fat and high level of omega-3 fat intake.

Look at the craze of the Atkins or the South Beach diets. These are diets based on restoring some sense of balance to the diets of Americans. Obviously, these are extreme examples. The Atkins diet is a high protein diet that can itself create imbalances and problems [634]. But simply reducing carb intake, increasing amino acid intake through increased protein, and better choices of fat intake (increased omega-3 and reduction in omega-6/saturated/trans fats), will reduce inflammation and in many individuals will result in weight loss. The mechanism of action is restoration of macronutrient balance and a reduction in inflammation. A book entitled

the Gruppo Italiano per lo Studio della Sopravvivenza nell-Infarto Miocardico (GISSI)-Prevenzione. Circulation. Apr 23 2002;105(16):1897-903.

631  Kris-Etherton PM, Harris, WS, Appel LJ. AHA Scientific statement: Fish Consumption, Fish oil, Omega-3 fatty acids, and cardiovascular disease. Circulation. 2002;106:2747-2757.

632  Chan DC, Watts GF, Mori TA, Barrett HR, Redgrave TG, Beilin LJ. Randomized controlled trial of the effect of n-3 fatty acid supplementation on the metabolism of apolipoprotein B-100 and chylomicron remnants in men with visceral obesity. Am J Clin Nutr. 2003;77:300-307.

633  Cote S et al. Very high concentrations of n-3 fatty acids in peri- and postmenopausal Inuit women from Greenland. Int J Circumpolar Health. 2004;63(2):298-301.

634  Metges CC, Barth CA. Metabolic consequences of a high dietary-protein intake in adulthood: assessment of the available evidence. J Nutr. Apr 2000;130(4):886-9.

*Inflammation Nation* by Floyd H. Chilton, touched on the impact of imbalanced fats, bad fat intake, and inflammation in the typical American diet.

Another way to reduce inflammation through diet is to reduce inflammatory foods. These foods will be unique to each individual and will often include foods that would typically be considered healthy. For example, my eldest daughter (beautiful as she is), has a food sensitivity to oranges. Oranges are healthy. Just not for my daughter. When my daughter eats oranges her lips swell, her abdomen hurts, and she feels tired. This is an inflammatory response. Remember the cardinal symptoms of inflammation? As previously discussed in the chapter on nutrition, this is not a food allergy in the classic sense of the word–such as found in a peanut allergy. However, it is an inflammatory response just the same (review the chapter on nutrition to review the testing involved). An inflammatory response that disrupts metabolism is an inflammatory response that leads to dysfunction, decreased metabolic performance, and to disease.

The latest addition to the inflammatory diet mix is GMOs. GMO is short for genetically modified foods. The perfect example of a GMO food is what some have referred to as the "Frankenfish". This is a salmon that is significantly larger than it's natural counterpart due to its genetic manipulation. I was recently in the grocery store and was walking through the fruit and vegetable section and was amazed at the size of the apples. They were like small watermelons. They were huge and they were genetically modified.

Bigger is better is the philosophy of GMOs. My reply to that statement is–in most cases it is not.

What is the big deal with GMO foods? GMO foods have been shown to increase inflammation signaling [635] [636]. In rat studies, GMO foods have been suggested to increase cancer. Except for recent research out of Europe, there is little scientific data on the long-term effects of GMOs. The problem with GMO research is that the majority of the research has been animal studies. No studies have looked at outcomes 90 days, except for Gilles-Eric Seralini. Seralini followed rats exposed to GMO maize (corn) for 2 years [637] and found increased incidence of mammary tumors. Another example is found with wheat. The fantastic book, *Wheat Belly*, showed how the wheat of today is simply not the wheat our bodies are familiar with. It is not even the same genetic plant structure. The impact? Try not eating GMO wheat and then adding it back in. Your body will let you know the impact–inflammation.

We just don't know the impact of GMO foods on our bodies and that is the problem. As a physician, that is not at all comforting to me. It is one thing for the government and the food industry to conduct experiments on me at 42 (though I would protest that). It is quite another to do so on my children and the children in America. The current estimates are that there are 10,000 food and chemical additives in our food supply. That amounts to about 14 lbs of chemical additives. These additives are toxins in most cases and are one of the factors for the growing obesity problem today [638].

---

635  Dutton A, Klein H, Romeis J, Bigler F. Uptake of Bt-toxin by herbivores feeding on transgenic maize and consequences for th epredator Chrysoperia carnea. Ecol Entomol. 2002;27:441-7.

636  Verma C, Nanda S, Singh RK, Singh RB, Mishra S. A review on impacts of genetically modified food on human health. The Open Nutraceuticals Journal. 2011;4:3-11.

637  Seralin GE et al. Long term toxicity of a roundup herbicide and a roundup tolerant genetically modified maize. Food and Chemical Toxicology. Nov 2012;50(11):4221-4231.

638  Baillie-Hamilton PF. Chemical Toxins: A hypothesis to explain the global obesity epidemic. J Alt Comp Med. 2002;8(2):185-192.

Here is the scenario I expect to play out. After about 20-30 years of testing on the general public, our kids included, the studies will be closed and the results will be published. The results of 20-30 years of GMO foods in the diets of Americans will be discussed amongst all of the media. Experts will be marched out on every network and asked why we didn't see the negative health effects of GMO foods coming. This will be just another crisis. The call will be for more government intervention. The problem is that government intervention caused the problem to begin with by getting in bed with the food industry. The results of an adulterated food supply are already evident in the current obesity problem. Why do we need to add to it with GMO?

If inflammation cannot be reduced through a balance in macronutrients, a balance in fat intake, the removal of inflammatory foods, or the elimination of GMO foods, then supplementation is the next step. NF-kappaB is one of the primary mechanisms by which inflammation signaling is produced. There are many good natural NF-kappaB inhibitors that can be used in a good natural supplement regimen. Appendix A presents them one by one.

The answers in how to resolve inflammation is to look to the body. I know that seems simplified, but that is the best roadmap. Health is a road map. Each individuals inflammatory pathway is different. Thus their roadmap for inflammation resolution should be nothing other than unique. This should come as no surprise as we are each created wonderfully unique. But this has been one of the pitfalls of medicine today–the attempt to treat through a one size-fits-all approach. This is not founded in reality. It is founded in convenience. It is easier and more convenient to treat 40 patients daily the same way. It takes time and effort to analyze and create customized treatment plans for each individual.

The first step in inflammation reduction is weight loss. If you are one of the 67% that are either overweight or obese, you have to lose weight to reduce inflammation. Remember that fat is a hormone and inflammatory producing organ. Fat is not innate. It is very active. That is why obesity is associated with so many diseases. So, if you are overweight, your pathway for inflammation reduction must come through weight loss. If you have hormone problems and you are overweight, you must achieve weight loss as a part of your pathway to hormone balance. If you are overweight, Health can only be achieved through weight loss.

There are plenty of natural solutions to help the body on its road to health and wellness (in this case the battle against inflammation) that are supported in the scientific literature. Many would say that there is no scientific data to support "natural" therapies (Appendix A disproves that argument). One can tell a lie over and over again and over time many begin to believe the lie as truth. That does not negate the fact the lie is indeed a lie and the truth stands.

So, look to the body to "go to the mattresses" on inflammation. But in this battle, we want solutions. Solutions based in causation. No band-aids. Band-aids just kick the can down the road. In our government, we see where that philosophy has gotten us. Unfortunately, we have become a "kick-the-can down the road" society. It is easier and requires less effort, but it has also gotten us where we are today–no solutions, just more problems.

On to solutions!

# APPENDIX A

I heavily reference these supplements to show that those of us in the alternative medicine, complementary medicine, integrative medicine, functional medicine, or natural medicine (or whatever one chooses to call it) are merely following science. It is not hard to find it. Just google it. I did. Somehow the critics can't.

Vitamin D

Vitamin D is a powerful anti-inflammatory. Vitamin D is naturally provided through sun exposure. This is why we all need some sun exposure without sunscreen. You can just feel you spirits rise with sun exposure. That is the effects of vitamin D. It is wonderful! Of course, if sun exposure exceeds 30 minutes, use some skin protection, but be wary of the ingredients of the sunscreen.

Low vitamin D is associated with increased inflammation [639]. Low vitamin D results in an increase in inflammation because vitamin D itself inhibits inflammation signaling through several mecha-

---

639  Peterson CA, Heffernan ME. Serum tumor necrosis factor-alpha concentrations are negatively correlated with serum 25(OH)D concentrations in healthy women. J Inflammation;2008;5:10.

nisms. First, Vitamin D increases T-regulatory cells [640]. T-regulatory cells are now considered one of the primary regulators of the immune response [641]. Vitamin D decreases NF-KappaB activity by increasing IkappaBalpha levels. It is the release of NF-kappaB from IkappaBalpha in the cytosol of the cell that activates NF-kappaB. IkappaBalpha upregulation decreases the nuclear translocation of NF-kappaB and thus reduces the activity of NF-kappaB [642]. Vitamin D has also been shown to inhibit the inflammatory signaling of monocytes/macrophages stimulated by LPS [643] through gene activation of MKP-1.

Vitamin D supplementation needs to be with D3. Dosing of Vitamin D3 is based on the individual level of the client. So check with your medical provider. Most dosing I use is between the range of 5,000 to 10,000 IU daily. However, this depends on the individual.

## Resveratrol

Ahh.... the benefits of red wine. Red wine and the infamous resveratrol. The reason so many of us justify the consumption of wine (guilty as charged). But, resveratrol comes through in the health benefits. Resveratrol is classified as a phenol. Resveratrol inhibits NF-kappaB [644] itself. But resveratrol also inhibits TNF-

640 Prietl B et al. Vitamin D supplementation increases circulating regulatory T cells in apparently healthy subjects: Vitamin D treatment for autoimmune diseases? Israel Medical Association Journal. March 2010;12(3):136-139.

641 Vignali DAA, Collison LW, Workman CJ. How regulatory T cells work. Nat Rev Immunol. July 2008;(7):523-532.

642 Cohen-Lahav M, Shany S, Tobvin D, Chaimovitz C, Couvdevani A. Vitamin D decreases NFkappaB activity by increasing IkappaBalpha levels. Nephrol Dial Transplant. Apr 2006;21(4):889-97.

643 Zhang Y, Leung DY, Richers BN, Liu Y, Remigio LK, Riches DW, Goleva E. Vitamin D inhibits monocyte/macrophage proinflammatory cytokine production by targeting MAPK phospatase-1. J Immunol. Mar 2012;188(5):2127-35.

644 Holmes-McNary M, Baldwin (Jr) AS. Chemopreventive properties of trans-resveratrol are associated with inhibition of acativation of the IkB kinase. Cancer Res.

alpha stimulated NF-kappaB signaling [645] [646] in fat tissue and resveratrol inhibits IL-1beta stimulated activation of NF-kappaB [647].

The dosing of resveratrol is between 50 and 100 mg daily in supplement form. You can use red wine as a part of your health regimen for resveratrol support, but you would have to drink a lot of red wine to get to this level, so don't try. Do I have a glass of red wine most days? The answer is yes, because red wine has been shown to increase Testosterone levels [648] which has been shown to decrease inflammation in men.

So, how much resveratrol is in a glass of wine? One glass of wine will provide approximately 0.2 to 2 mg [649] [650]. Compared to the dosing in supplement form, you better be prepared to drink a lot of wine. The goal is balance. When a higher dosage than is provided for in a glass of wine is needed, resveratrol in supplement form is preferred.

## Omega-3

Who hasn't heard of the health benefits of fish oil. Remember that old wives tale of cod liver oil? There is science in many of those

2000;60:3477-3483.

645 Gonzales AM, Orlando RA. Curcumin and resveratrol inhibit nuclear factor-kappaB-mediated cytokine expression in adipocytes. Nutrition Metabolism. 2008;5:17.

646 Manna SK, Mukhopadhyah A, Aggarwal BB. Resveratrol suppresses TNF-induced activation of nuclear transcription factors NF-kappaB, activator protein-1, and apoptosis: potential role of reactive oxygen intermediates and lipid peroxidation. J Immunol. Jun 15 2000;164(12):6509-19.

647 Busch F, Mobasheri A, Shaya P, Lueders C, Stahlmann R, Shakibaei M. Resveratrol modulates IL-1beta-induces PI3K and NF-KappaB signaling pathways in human tenocytes. J Biol Chem. Nov 2 2012;287(45):38050-63.

648 Jenkinson C, Petroczi A, Naughton DP. Red wine and component flavonoids inhibit UGT2B17 in vitro. Nutrional Journal. 2012;11:67.

649 Fremont L. Biological effects of resveratrol. Life Sci. 2000;66(8):663-673.

650 Siemann EH, Creasey LL. Concentration of the phytoalexin resveratrol in wine. Am J Enol Vitic. 1992;43(1):49-52.

old tales. Omega-3 inhibits NF-kappaB through inhibition of lkappaB phosphylation which inhibits the disassociation of lkappaB and NF-KappaB[651]. As a result, omega-3 inhibits the production of pro-inflammatory cytokins [652]. Omega-3's even inhibit cycloxygenase enzyme activity, which is responsible for the production of inflammatory prostaglandins [653].

Most dose too low with Omega-3. The inuit eskimoes have been estimated to take in an estimated 8+ grams daily through their diet. First, eat more fish. The best fish choice is the fresh, wild caught fish that is of the non-farm raised variety. The great Northwest salmon varieties and Halibut are great additions to any diet. Try to avoid fish high on the food chain as they accumulate mercury from other fish. Farm raised fish are also higher in mercury content. If you are one of those people that just don't like fish and other seafood items, then oral supplementation is the way to go. Most under dose with regards to omega-3 supplementation. Dosing is always best done under the care of a medical provider that is familiar with the research on omega-3. I typically dose omega-3 in the range of 3,000 mg to 6,000 mg daily. I may even dose higher based on test results. To much omega-3 can have a blood thinning effect, so be on the watch if you are taking other blood thinners. Definitely let your doctor know of your omega-3 intake if you are on blood thinners.

---

651  Novak TE, Babcock TA, Jho DH, Helton WS, Espat NJ. NF-kappaB inhibition by omega-3 fatty acids modulates LPS-stimulated macrophages TNF-alpha transcription. Am J Physiol Lung Cell Mol Physiol. Jan 2003;284(1):L84-9.

652  Kang JX, Weylandt KH. Modulation of inflammatory cytokines by omega-3 fatty acids. Subcell Biochem. 2008;49:133-43.

653  Martinez-Micaelo N, Gaonzalez-Abuin N, Terra X, Richart C, Ardevol A, Pinent M, Blay M. Omega-3 docosahexaenoic acid and procyanidins inhibit cyclo-oxygenase activity and attenuate NF-kappaB activation through a p105/p50 regulatory mechanism in macrophage inflammation. Biochem J. Jan 15 2012;441(2):653-63.

# Curcumin

Who doesn't like a little spice in their food? Having lived in Louisiana, I know this first hand. They put cayenne pepper, Louisiana hot sauce, and Tobasco on everything! Curcumin is one of the main components of the Indian spice Turmeric. Another polyphenol. Turmeric has been a component of Ayurvedic medicine for thousands of years.

Curcumin has several anti-inflammatory properties. Curcumin blocks inflammatory cytokine generating NF-kappaB activity [654] [655] [656] and down regulates cyclooxygenase 2 (COX-2) and metalloproteinase-9 (MMP-9) [657] in those with arthritis. Additionally, curcumin has been shown to have numerous benefits in other inflammatory disease like cancer (inhibiting initiation [658] and proliferation [659] of cancer cells), and in ulcerative colitis [660]. Most of this occurs through NF-kappaB inhibition.

654 Jobin C, Bradham CA, Russo MP, Juma B, Narula AS, Brenner DA, Sartor RB. Curcumin blocks cytokine-mediated NF-kappaB activation and proinflammatory gene expression by inhibiting inhibitory factor I-kappaB kinase activity. J Immunol. Sep 15 1999;163(6):3474-83.

655 Poylin V, Fareed MU, O'Neal P, Alamdari N, Reilly N, Menconi M, Hasselgren PO. The NF-kappaB inhibitor curcumin blocks sepsis-induced muscle proteolysis. Mediators Inflamm. 2008;2008:317851.

656 Plummer SM et al. Inhibition of cyclo-oxygenase 2 expression in colon cells by the chemopreventive agent curcumin involves inhibition of NF-kappaB activation via the NIK/IKK signaling complex. Oncogene. 199;18(44):6013-6020.

657 Shakibaei M, John T, Schulze-Tanzil G, Lehmann I, Mobasheri A. Suppression of NF-kappaB activation by curcumin leads to inhibition of expression of cyclo-oxygenase-2 and matrix metalloproteinase-9 in human articular chondrocytes: Implications for the treatment of osteoarthritis. Biochem Pharmacol. May 1 2007;73(9):1434-45.

658 Huang MT, Wang ZY, Georgiadis CA, Laskin JD, Conney AH. Inhibitory effects of curcumin on tumore initiation by benzo[a]pyrene and 7,12-dimethylbenz[a] anthracene. Carcinogenesis. 1992;13:2183-6.

659 Conney AH et al. Inhibitory effect of curcumin and some related dietary compounds on tumor promotion and arachidonic acid metabolism in mouse skin. Adv Enzyme Regul. 1991;31:385-96.

660 Hanai H et al. Curcumin maintenance therapy for ulcerative colitis: randomized, multicenter, double-blind, placebo controlled trial. Clin Gastroenterol Hepatol. 2006;4:1502-1506.

Like many of these natural anti-inflammatories, just add it into your diet. Spice it up. Use curcumin as a new spice in your cooking. Or just eat you some delicious Indian food, particularly curry. But, if that doesn't fit your style, there is curcumin in supplemental form. However, understand that curcumin has poor oral bioavailability [661], thus higher dosages are required to achieve benefits outside the gastrointestinal tract. For that reason, I dose curcumin in the range of 2-4 grams daily for the gastrointestinal problems and 4-8 grams daily for systemic problems.

## Boswellia

This is one of my favorites. You may know it better as Frankincense. Frankincense is a resin that can be distilled into an essential oil, but it is not just for aroma therapy. There are several types of Boswellia. There is Boswellia sacra, Boswellia carteri, Boswellia frereana, and Boswellia serrata to name a few and not all contain the same level of boswellic acid. Some species, despite their name actually have none.

Not only does it smell great, but it has tremendous health benefits. Remember that it was one of the 3 gifts to Jesus. It wasn't just about the symbolism (Frankincense, gold, and myrrh were extremely valuable), but there were also tremendous health benefits to baby Jesus.

There are several anti-inflammatory actions of Boswellia. Boswellia has been shown to decrease inflammation through inhibition of 5-lipoxygenase [662], inhibition of prostaglandin E2 synthase-1 [663], and

---

661  Sharma RA, Gescher AJ, Steward WP. Curcumin: the story so far. Eur J Cancer. 2005;41(13):1955-1968.

662  Ammon HP. Boswellic acids in chronic inflammatory diseases. Planta Med. Oct 2006;72(2):1100-16.

663  Siemoneit U et al. Inhibition of microsomal prostaglandin E2 synthase-1 as a molecular basis for the anti-inflammatory actions of boswellic acids from frankincense. Br J Pharmacol. Jan 2011;162(1):147-62.

inhibition of NF-kappaB expression [664] [665] [666]. In addition, Boswellia has shown to provide benefits in breast cancer [667], brain cancer [668], leukemia [669], meningioma [670], inflammatory bowel disease [671], and osteoarthritis [672].

Dosing? The great thing about Boswellia is it is available in the essential oil form. There is no standardized dosage. This can be applied through the skin or can be placed in capsules and ingested. The best benefits come from Boswellia sacra and should be applied to the skin/effected area daily. As previously stated, it is best to take Boswellia under the care from a provider familiar with the medicinal use and side effects of Boswellia.

---

664 Takada Y, Ichikawa H, Badmaev, Aggarwal BB. Acetyl-11-keto-beta-boswellic acid potentiates apoptosis, inhibits invasion, and abolishes osteoclastogenesis by suppressing NF-kappa B and NF-kappa B-regulated gene expression. J Immunol. Mar 1 2006; 176(5):3127-40.

665 Cuaz-Perolin C et al. Antiinflammatory and antiatheogenic effects of the NF-kappaB inhibitor acetyl-11-keto-beta-boswellic acid in LPS-challenged ApoE-/- mice. Arterioscler Thromb Vasc Biol. Feb 2008;28(2):272-7.

666 Syrovets T, Buchele B, Krauss C, Laumonnier Y, Simmet T. Acetyl-boswellic acids inhibit lipopolysaccharide-mediated TNF-alpha induction in monocytes by direct interaction with lkappaB kinases. J Immunol. Jan 1 2005;174(1):498-506.

667 Suhaii MM et al. Boswellia sacra essential oil induces tumor cell-specific apoptosis and suppresses tumor aggressiveness in human breast cancer cells. BMC Complement Altern Med. Dec 15 2011;11:129.

668 Reising K et al. Determination of boswellic acids in brain and plasma by high-performance liquid chromatography/tandem mass spectrometry. Anal Chem. 2005;77:6640-6645.

669 Jing Y et al. Boswellic acid acetate induces differentiation and apoptosis in leukemia cell lines. Leukemia Research. 1999;23:43-50.

670 Park YS et al. Cytotoxic action of acetyl-11-keto-boswellic acid (AKBA) on meningioma cells. Planta Med. 2002;68:397-401.

671 Joos SS, Rosemann TT et al. Use of complementary and alternative medicine in Germany–a survey of patients with inflammatory bowel disease. BMC complementary and Alternative Medicine. 2006;6:19.

672 Kimmatkar N et al. Efficacy and tolerability of Boswellia serrata extract in treatment of osteoarthritis of knee–a randomized double-blind placebo controlled trial. Phytomedicine. 2003;10:3-7.

## EGCG

EGCG is the most abundant catechin found in tea, particularly green tea. Many have heard of the health benefits of green tea. EGCG is the active antioxidant behind the benefits of green tea.

EGCG has been shown to provide many benefits. EGCG has been shown to protect against cancer [673], reduce elevated cholesterol [674], protect against oxidative damage [675], protect against cardiovascular disease [676], protect against endothelial dysfunction [677], aid in type II Diabetes [678] treatment, and aid in weight loss [679] [680]. Of course, EGCG decreases inflammation (cytokines and chemokines) through inhibition of the phosphorylation of MAPKs p38, JNK, AP-1, and of course the all important NF-kappaB [681].

673  Singh BN, Shankar S, Srivastava RK. Green tea catechin, epigallocatechin-3-gallate (EGCG): mechanisms, perspectives and clinical applications. Biochem Pharmacol. Dec 15 2011;82(12):1807-21.

674  Koo Si, Noh SK. Green tea as inhibitor of the intestingal absorption of lipids: potential mechanism for its lipid-lowering effect. J Nutr Biochem. 2007;18:179-183.

675  Luo H et al. Phas IIa chemoprevention trial of green tea polyphenols in high-risk individuals of liver cancer: modulation of urinary excretion of green tea polyphenols and 8-hydroxydeoxyguanosine. Carcinogenesis. 2006;27:262-268.

676  Shimada et al. Oolong tea increases plasma adiponectin levels and low-density lipoprotein particle size in patients with coronary artery disease. Diabetes Res Clin Pract. 2004;65:227-234.

677  Kim W et al. Effect of green tea consumpton on endothelial function and circulating endothelial progenitor cells in chronic smokers. Circ. 2006;J70:1052-1057.

678  Hosoda K, Wang MF, Liao ML, Chuang CK, Iha M, Elevidence B, Yamamoto S. Antihyperglycemic effect of oolong tea in type 2 diabetes. Diabetes Care. 2003;26:1714-1718.

679  Hase TK, Meguro S, Takeda Y, Takahashi H. Anti-obesity effects of tea catechins in humans. J Olea Sci. 2001;50:599-605.

680  Tsuchida T, Itakura H, Nakamura H. Reduction of body fat in humans by long-term ingestion of catechins. Prog Med. 2002;22:2189-2203.

681  Cavet ME et al. Anti-inflammatory and anti-oxidative effects of the green tea polyphenol epigallocatechin gallate in human corneal epithelial cells. Mol Vis. 2011;17:533-542.

EGCG is easiest consumed via green tea. Studies [682] have shown that dosing in the range of 5-6 cups of green tea daily is appropriate. If you don't like green tea or 5-6 cups of green tea is to much, then 200-300 mg of EGCG through oral supplementation is a good alternative.

## Quercetin

Quercetin is a bioflavoniod that is derived from oak forest. Quercetin is the most prevalent bioflavonoid in nature and is a powerful antioxidant that is commonly found in red wine, green tea, fruits and vegetables.

Quercetin has multiple anti-inflammatory effects. Quercetin reduces inflammatory cytokines (TNF-alpha, IL-6, IL-1beta), decreases cycloxygenase-2 expression (COX-2), decreases phosphorylated JNK and c-Jun [683], and decreases NF-kappaB activity [684] [685]. The final result of the effects of Quercetin is the inhibition of inflammatory signaling.

In addition, Quercetin has been shown to have anti-cancer properties in cell and animal models [686], has been shown to aid

---

682 Wolfram S. Effects of green tea and EGCG on cardiovascular and metabolic health. J Am Coll Nutr. Aug 2007;26(4):373S-388S.

683 Overman A, Chuang CC, McIntosh M. Quercetin attenuates inflammation in human macrophages and adipocytes exposed to macrophage-conditioned media. Int J Obes; Jan 2011;35:1165-72.

684 Granado-Serrano AB, Martin MA, Bravo L, Goya L, Ramos S. Quercetin modulates NF-kappaB and AP-1/JNK pathways to induce cell death in human hepatoma cells. Nutr Cancer. 2010/62(3):390-401.

685 Comalada M et al. In vivo quercitrin anti-inflammatory effect involves release of quercetin, whihc inhibits inflammation through down-regulation of the NF-kappaB pathway. Eur J Immunol. 2005;35:584-592.

686 Bibellini L et al. Quercetin and Cancer chemoprevention. Evidence-Based Complementary and Alternative Medicine. 2011;2011:591356.

prostatitis [687], and has been shown to benefit allergic asthma [688]. It stands to reason that Quercetin can benefit any individual suffering from inflammation or oxidative stress.

The dosage of Quercetin is not standard and is variable for the treatment. I dose Quercetin in the range of 500 to 1,000 mg without any side effects. This should be taken in 3 divided doses daily.

## Astaxanthin

Astaxanthin is a relative newcomer and is a very hot topic today. Astaxanthin is a natural carotenoid found in shrimp, lobster, salmon, and trout. Astaxanthin gives these crustaceans and fish their characteristic red color. Astaxanthin is a powerful antioxidant [689]. Astaxanthin has been shown to inhibit breast tumor growth [690], has been shown to decrease bacterial load and inflammation in H. pylori infection [691], to provide cardiovascular protection, decrease lipid peroxidation and decrease thrombosis

---

687  Shoskes DA, Zeitlin SI, Shahed A, Rajfer J. Quercetin in men with category III chronic prostatitis: a preliminary prospective, double-blind, placebo-controlled trial. Urology. Dec 1999;54(6):960-3.

688  Joskova M, Franova S, Sadionova V. Acute bronchodilator effect of quercetin in experimental allergic asthma. Bratisl Lek Listy. 2011;112(1):9-12.

689  Park JS, Chyun JH, Kim YK, Line LL, Chew BP. Astaxanthin decreased oxidative stress and inflammation and enhanced immune response in humans. Nutrition Metabolism. 2010;7:18.

690  Chew BP, Park JS, Wong MW, Wong TS. A comparison of the anticancer activities of dietary B-carotene, canthaxanthin and astaxanthin in mice in vivo. Anticancer Res. 1999;19:1849-1853.

691  Bennedsen M, Wang X, Willen R, Wadstrom T, Andersen LP. Treatment of H. pylori infected mice with antioxidant astaxanthin reduces gastric inflammation, bacterial load and modulates cytokine release by splenocytes. Immunol Lett. 1999;70:185-189.

through reduction in oxidative stress [692] [693] [694] and inflammation [695] [696] [697] [698]. All these benefits were shown in vitro and in animal models. Astaxanthin inhibits inflammation through the inhibition of NF-kappaB activation [699].

Dosing of astaxanthin is variable and is based on safety, bioavailability and effect studies. The ranges in these studies range from 4 mg to 100 mg per day. I typically recommend 20 to 40 mg daily, but this varies based on the purpose of action. I don't usually dose astaxanthin as high individually because I combine astaxanthin with other antioxidants.

One caveat about astaxanthin. There is some suggestion that astaxanthin inhibits 5-alpha reductase [700] in men.

692   O'Connor I, O'Brien NM. Modulation of UVA light-induced oxidative stress by beta-carotene, lutein and astaxanthin in cultured fibroblasts. J Dermatol Sci. 1988;16:226-230.

693   Iwamoto T et al. Inhibition of low-density lipoprotein oxidation by astaxanthin. J Atheroscler Thromb. 2007;7:216-222.

694   Karppi J, Rissanen TH, Nyyssonen K, Kaikkonen J, Olsson AG, Voutilainen S, SalonenJT. Effects of astaxanthin supplementation on lipid peroxidation. Int JVitam Nutr Res. 2007;77:3-11.

695   Ohgami K et al. Effects of astaxanthin on lipopolysaccharide-induced inflammation in vitro and in vivo. Invest Ophthalmol Vis Sci. 2003;44:2694-2701.

696   Lee SJ et al. Astaxanthin inhibits nitric oxide production and inflammatory gene expression by suppressing I(kappa)B kinase-dependent NF-kappaB activation. Mol Cells. 2003;16:97-105.

697   Nakano M et al. Effect of astaxanthin in combination with alpha-tocopherol or ascorbic acid against oxidative damage in diabetic ODS rats. J Nutr Sci Vitaminol (Tokyo). 2008;54:329-334.

698   Choi SK, Park YS, Choi DK, Chang HI. Effects of astaxanthin on the production of NO and the expression of COX-2 and iNOS in LPS-stimulated BV2 microglial cells. J Microbiol Biotechnol. 2008;18:1990-1996.

699   Seon-Jin Lee et al. Astaxanthin Inhibits Nitric Oxide Production and Inflammatory gene expression by suppressing IkB Kinase-dependent NF-kappaB Activation. Mol Cells. 2003;16(1):97-105.

700   Anderson ML. A preliminary investigation of the enzymatic inhibitio of 5alpha-reduction and growht of prostatic carcinoma cell lin LNCap-FGC by natural astaxanthin and Saw Palmetto Lipid extract in vitro. J Herb Pharmacother. 2005;5(1):17-26.

## Sulforaphane

Sulforaphane Is a natural isothiocyanate found in crucifer-ous vegetables like broccoli, cabbage, and brussel sprouts. Sulforaphane is a potent stimulator of phase II detoxification [701], sulforaphane has been shown to have anti-cancer proper-ties[702] in breast cancer [703] [704], prostate cancer [705], colon cancer [706], and in pancreatic cancer [707] to name a few. Sulforaphane inhibits inflammation through direct NF-kappaB inhibition[708], through inhibition of Prostaglandin E2 [709], and indirectly through Nrf2 activation [710]. The point is, sulforphane provides great benefit to many states of disease and dysfunction, but especially to inflam-

701 Shen G et al. Chemoprevention of familial adenomatous polposis by natural dietary compounds sulforaphane and dibenzoylmethane alone and in combina-tion in ApcMin/+ mouse. Cancer Res. 2007;67:9937-9944.

702 Zhang Y, Kensler TW, Cho CG, Posner GH, Talalay P. Anticarcinogenic activities of sulforaphane and structurally related synthetic norbornyl isothiocyanates. Proc Natl Acad Sci U S A. 1994;91:3147-3150.

703 Johnston N. Sulforaphane halts breast cancer growth. Drug Discovery Today. 2004;9(21):908.

704 Pledgie-Tracy A, Sobolewski MD, Davidson NE. Sulforaphane induces cell type-spe-cific apoptosis in human breast cancer cell lines. Mol Cancer Ther. Mar 2007;6(3):1013-21.

705 Singh SV et al. Sulforaphane-induced cell death in human prostate cancer cells is initiated by reactive oxygen species. Journal of Biological Chemistry. May 20 2005;280:19911-19924.

706 Frydoonfar HR, McGrath DR Spigelman AD. Sulforaphane inhibits growth of a colon cancer cell line. Colorectal Dis. Jan 2004;6(1):28-31.

707 Li Y et al. Sulforaphane inhibits pancreatic cancer through disrupting Hsp90-p50(Cdc37) complex and direct interactions with amino acids residues of Hsp90. J Nutr Biochem. Dec 2012;23(12):1617-26.

708 Heiss E et al. Nuclear Factor kB is a molecular target for sulforaphane-medi-ated Anti-inflammatory mechanisms. Journal of Biological Chemistry. Aug 2001;276(34):32008-32015.

709 Zhou J, Joplin DG, Cross JV, Templeton DJ. Sulforaphane inhibits prostaglandin E2 synthesis by suppressing microsomal prostaglandin E synthase 1. PLoS One. 2012;7(11):e49744. doi:10.1371/journal.pone.0049744.

710 Lin W, Wu RT, Wu T, Khor TO, Want H, Kong AN. Sulforaphane suppressed LPS-induced inflammation in mouse peritoneal macrophages through Nrf2 depen-dent pathway. Biochem Pharmacol. Oct 2008;76(8):967-73.

mation. Remember, inflammation is a prerequisite for cancer through promoting cell growth [711] and inhibiting programmed cell death.

How to dose sulforaphane? One of the best methods is to simply eat sulforaphane through the broccoli, cabbage, brussel sprouts, and the like. Mom had it right, "eat your vegetables". For those of you non-vegetable eaters, then sulforaphane is available in oral supplementation. The exact bioavailability of sulforapahane is unknown. That being said, I use a sulforaphane dosage of 200-400 mg daily in divided doses as a start. High dosing should be under the care of a provider aware of the physiologic actions of sulforaphane. I recommend that this be done above and beyond regular veggie intake.

## Vitamin C

Vitamin C is one of my absolute favorites. Vitamin C is of course a vitamin and a powerful antioxidant. Vitamin C is one of the more studied antioxidants around. Vitamin C is interesting in that humans lack the endogenous capacity to make vitamin C, so we must get vitamin C through our diet. Vitamin C is great orally, but has its limitation due to GI upset. This seems to occur in the 5,000 to 10,000 mg range.

Vitamin C has been shown to be a useful aid in the treatment of many disease states. Vitamin C has been shown to improve vasodilation and improve blood flow [712] [713]. Vitamin C has been shown to aid in

---

711 Steel VE, Hawk ET, Viner JL, Lubet RA. Mechanisms and applications of non-steroidal anti-inflammatory drugs in the chemoprevention of cancer. Mutat Res. 2003;523-524:137-144.

712 Gokce N et al. Long-term ascorbic acid administration reverses enothelial vasomotor dysfunction in patients with coronary artery disease. Circulation. 1999;99(25):3234-3240.

713 Versari D, Daghini E, Virdis A, Ghiadoni L, Taddei S. Endothelium-dependent contractions and endothelial dysfunction in human hypertension. Br J Pharmacol. 2009;157(4):527-536.

lowering blood pressure [714]. Vitamin C in high doses has been shown to be useful adjuncts in cancer treatment [715 716 717 718]. Vitamin C has even been shown to reduce the common cold [719 720] through vitamin C's immune stimulatory effect [721 722 723 724 725 726]. And of course, vitamin C has been shown to reduce inflammation in individuals with cancer. A 2012 study found a reduction of inflammatory cancer biomarkers in prostate cancer, breast cancer, bladder cancer, pancreatic cancer, lung cancer, thyroid cancer, skin cancer and Lymphoma [727].

714 Duffy SJ et al. Treatment of hypertension with ascorbic acid. Lancet. 1999;354(9195):2048-2049.

715 Padayatty SJ et al. Vitamin C pharmacokinetics: implications for oral and intravenous use. Ann Intern Med. 2004;140(7):533-537.

716 Cameron E, Pauling L. Supplemental ascorbate in the supportive treatment of cancer: prolongation of survival times in terminal human cancer. Proce Natl Acad Sci U S A. 1976;73(10):3685-3689.

717 Chen Q et al. Pharmacologic ascorbic acid concentrations selectively kill cancer cells: action as a pro-drug to deliver hydrogen peroxide to tissues. Proc Natl Acad Sci U S A. 2005;102(38):13604-13609.

718 Riordan HD et al. A pilot clinical study of continuous intravenous ascorbate in terminal cancer patients. P R Health Sci J. 2005;24(4):269-276.

719 Pauling LC. Vitamin C and the common cold. San Francisco: W.H. Freeman;1970.

720 Douglas RM, Hemila H, D'Souza R, Chalker EB, Treacy B. Vitamin C for preventing and treating the common cold. Cochrane Database Syst Rev. 2004(4):CD000980.

721 Prinz W, Bortz R, Bregin B, Hersch M. The effect of ascorbic acid supplementation on some parameters of the human immunological defense system. Int J Vitam Nutr Res. 1977;47(3):248-257.

722 Vallance S. Relationships between ascorbic acid and serum proteins of the immune system. Br Med J. 1977;2(6084):437-438.

723 Kennes B, Dumont I, Brohee D, Hubert C, Neve P. Effect of vitamin C supplements on cell-mediated immunity in old people. Gerontology. 1983;29(5):305-310.

724 Panush RS, Delafuente JC, Katz P, Johnson J. Modulation of certain immunologic responses by vitamin C. III. Potentiation of in vitro and in vivo lymphocyte responses. Int J Vitamin Nutr Res Suppl. 1982;23:35-47.

725 Anderson R, Oosthuizen R, Maritz R, Theron A, Van Rensburg AJ. The effects of increasing weekly doses of ascorbate on certain cellular and humoral immune functions in normal volunteers. Am J Clin Nutr. 1980;33(1):71-76.

726 Anderson R. The immunostimulatory, antiinflammatory and anti-allergic properties of ascorbate. Adv Nutr Res. 1984;6:19-45.

727 Mikirova N, Casciari J, Rogers A, Taylor P. Effect of high-dose intravenous vitamin C on inflammation in cancer patients. J Transl Med. 2012;10:189.

Vitamin C has been shown to reduce oxidative stress and NF-kappaB activation in individuals with rheumatoid arthritis [728].

Dosing of Vitamin C is simple. Take as much as you can tolerate. As I stated above, most find this to be in the range of 5-10 grams daily through oral supplementation. The benefits of vitamin C in cancer were found in dosing above that which is tolerated orally and only found through IV dosing. In fact, Intravenous vitamin C is the only mode that has been show to raise blood levels of vitamin C [126]. The minimum dosage of daily vitamin C is 400 mg daily. The only potential side effect is a suggestion of increased risk of oxalate kidney stones. So, if you have a history of kidney stones, check with your medical provider.

## MSM

If you have any joint pain you are probably familiar with MSM. MSM is short for methylsulfonylmethane. It is a common component in joint pain supplements and has been shown to be beneficial in osteoarthritis [729] [730]. The evidence is not overwhelming, but benefit is seen without side effects. MSM has been shown to decrease inflammation through down regulation of NF-kappaB activity [731].

728  Mikirova N, Rogers A, Casciaria J, Taylor P. Effect of high dose intravenous ascorbic acid on the level of inflammation in patients with rheumatoid arthritis. Modern Research in Inflammation. 2012;1(2):26-32.

729  Debbi EM et al. Efficacy of methylsulfonylmethane supplementation on osteoarthritis of the knee: a randomized controlled study. BMC Complement Altern Med. Jun 27 2011;11:50.

730  Kim LS, Axelrod LJ, Howard P, Buratovich N, Waters RF. Efficacy of methylsulfonylmethan (MSM) in osteoarthritis pain of the knee: a pilot clinical trial. Osteoarthritis Cartilage. Mar 2006;14(3):286-94.

731  Kim YH, Kim DH, Lim H, Baek DY, Shin HK, Kim JK. The anti-inflammatory effects of methylsulfonylmethane on lipopolysaccharide-induced inflammation responses in murine macrophages. Biol Pharm Bull. Apr 2009;32(4):651-6.

Dosing is simple for MSM. Start at 500 mg and increase to 3,000 mg in divided daily doses. Studies have shown higher dosing for other conditions. These higher dosages should occur under the guidance of a provider familiar with MSM.

## Alpha Lipoic Acid

Alpha Lipoic Acid is one of my favorite supplements. Alpha Lipoic Acid is a naturally present compound. However, humans do not make Alpha Lipoic Acid. Alpha Lipoic Acid is a major component of the pyruvate dehydrogenase enzyme, which is involved in glycolysis.

Alpha Lipoic Acid has many benefits. Alpha Lipoic Acid is a powerful antioxidant [732] [733]. Alpha Lipoic Acid aids insulin in glucose uptake at the level of the GLUT4 receptor [734]. Intravenous Alpha Lipoic Acid has been shown to aid those suffering with peripheral neuropathy [735] [736]. Alpha Lipoic Acid increases glutathione production in in-vitro and in-vivo studies [737]. Alpha Lipoic Acid is a weak

732  Packer L, Witt EH, Tritschler HJ. Alpha-Lipoic acid as a biological antioxidant. Free Radic Biol Med. Aug 1995;19(2):227-50.

733  Neuroprotection by the metabolic antioxidant alpha-lipoic acid. Neuroprotection by the metabolic antioxidant alpha-lipoic acid. Free Radic Biol Med. 1997;22(1-2):359-78.

734  Konrad D, Somwar R, Sweeney G, Yaworsky K, Hayashi M, Ramlal T, Klip A. The antihyperglycemic drug alpha-lipoic acid stimulates glucose uptake via both GLUT4 translocation and GLUT4 activation: potential role of p38 mitogen-activated protein kinase in GLUT4 activation. Diabetes. Jun 2001;50(6):1464-71.

735  Mijnhout GS, Kollen BJ, Alkhalaf A, Kleefstra N, Bilo HJ. Alpha lipoic acid for symptomatic peripheral neuropathy in patients with diabetes: a meta-analysis of randomized controlled trials. Int J Endocrinol. 2012;2012:456279.

736  Ziegler D. Thiotic acid for patients with symptomatic diabetic polyneuropathy: a critical review. Treat Endocrinol. 2004;3(3):173-89.

737  Busse E, Zimmer G, Schopohl B, Kornhuber B. Influence of alpha-lipoic acid on intracellular glutathione in vitro and in vivo. Arzneimittelforschung. Jun 1992.42(6):829-31.

chelator [738]. And of course, Alpha Lipoic Acid inhibits inflammation [739] [740], primarily through NF-kappaB inhibition [741] [742].

Dosing of oral Alpha Lipoic Acid should be limited to 600 mg daily. Additional dosing should be under the care of a medical provider. Additionally, look for specialized physicians that can provide IV Alpha Lipoic Acid for peripheral neuropathy and additional benefits.

## Melatonin

Melatonin is an actual hormone. Melatonin is produced from the pineal gland. Melatonin is an indoleamine that is derived from the amino acid tryptophan. Melatonin is everywhere because many struggle to achieve good, restful sleep.

Melatonin is not just for sleep. Melatonin functions as an antioxidant [743]. Melatonin is proposed to play an anticancer role. High light exposure at night decreases melatonin production

---

738  Yamamoto et al. The antioxidant effect of DL-alpha-lipoic acid on copper-induced acute hepatitis in Long-Evans Cinnamon (LEC) rats. Free Radic Res. Jan 2001;34(1):69-80.

739  Odabasoglu F et al. Alpha-lipoic acid has anti-inflammatory and anti-oxidative properties: an experimental study in rats with carrageenan-induced acute and cotton pellet-induced chronic inflammations. Br J Nutr. Jan 2011;105(1):31-43.

740  Khabbazi T, Mahdavi R, Safa J, Pour-Abdollahi P. Effects of alpha-lipoic acid supplementation on inflammation, oxidative stress, and serum lipid profile levels on patients with end-state renal disease on hemodialysis. J Ren Nutr. Mar 2012;22(2):244-50.

741  Zhang WJ, Frei B. Alpha-lipoic acid inhibits TNF-alpha-induced NF-kappaB activation and adhesion molecule expression in human aortic endothelial cells. FASEB J. Nov 2001;15(13):2423-32.

742  Lee HA, Hughes DA. Alpha-lipoic acid modulates NF-kappaB activity in human monocytic cells by direct interaction with DNA. Exp Gerontol. Jan-Mar 2002;37(2-3):401-10.

743  Reiter RJ, Tan DX, Mayo JC, Sainz RM, Leon J, Czarnocki Z. Melatonin as an antioxidant: biochemical mechanisms and pathophysiological implicaitons in humans. Acta Biochim Pol. 2003;50(4):1129-46.

and increases breast cancer risk significantly [744]. The mechanism of melatonin's proposed anti-cancer effect is primarily through it's inhibition of inflammation. One mechanism of the proposed anticancer benefit is through the interference by melatonin in the estrogen signaling pathway. Melatonin directly inhibits estrogen receptor alpha [745] and if you remember from chapter 9, ER alpha is associated with a pro-growth and pro-inflammatory signaling. Melatonin also blocks intracellularly activated ER-alpha signaling [746]. Cancer cells use this receptor to grow through a pro-growth and pro-inflammatory environment. Melatonin also inhibits inflammation through modulation of Nrf-2 and NF-kappaB [747]. Melatonin has been shown to provide neuroprotection in diabetic neuropathy via the same mechanism [748]. Additionally, melatonin has been shown to reduce IL-6 and erythrocyte sedimentation rate (ESR) [749].

The over the counter dosing of melatonin varies. The standard dosing I recommend is 1 to 3 mg nightly. Higher dosing should be under the guide of a medical provider knowledgeable of the effects of melatonin. One caveat about melatonin. Melatonin can

---

744  Kloog I, Haim A, Stevens RB, Barchana M, Portnov BA. Light at night co-distributes with incident breast but not lung cancer in female population of Israel. Chronobiol Int. 2008;25(1):65-81.

745  Martinez-Campa C et al. Melatonin inhibits both ER alpha activation and breast cancer cell proliferation induced by a metalloestrogen cadmium. J Pineal Res. May 2006;40(4):291-6.

746  del Rio B et al. Melatonin, an endogenous specific inhibitor of estrogen receptor alpha via calmodulin. J Biol Chem. 2004;279(37):38294-38302.

747  Tripathi DN, Jena GB. Effect of melatonin on the expression of Nrf2 adn NF-kappaB during cyclophosphamide-induced urinary bladder injury in rat. J Pineal Res. May 2010;48(4):324-31.

748  Negi G, Kumar A, Sharma SS. Melatonin modulates neuroinflammation and oxidative stress in experimental diabetic neuropathy: effects on NF-kappaB and Nrf2 cascades. J Pineal Res. Mar 2011;50(2):124-31.

749  Lissoni P et al. Melatonin as a new possible anti-inflammatory agent. J Biol Regul Homeost Agents. 1997;11(4):157-159.

produce vivid dreams. So, if you have nightmares or vivid dreams already–be cautious.

## Cordyceps

Cordyceps is one of my favorites–particularily Cordyceps Sinensis. Cordyceps has been used by traditional Chinese and Tibetan medicine for thousands of years. Thousands of years of observation data is powerful evidence. It has been called the elixir of youth and longevity. Cordyceps is commonly known as a caterpillar fungus. That is always fun to explain. But, Cordyceps is actually a mushroom. Cordyceps was first discovered to be used by the Chinese women's 1984 olympic swim team to improve athletic performance. It has since been used by many others.

Cordyceps has many benefits, but cordyceps is a powerful inhibitor of inflammation. Cordyceps has been shown to have anti-tumor, anti-metastatic, immunomodulatory, antioxidant, insecticidal, antimicrobial, neuroprotective and renoprotective effects [750]. Cordyceps has also been shown to decrease inflammation. Cordyceps has been shown to reduce pulmonary inflammation by inhibiting NF-kappaB activity [751]. Specifically, Cordyceps has been shown to reduce LPS stimulated NO production, reduce NF-kappaB expression, reduce IkappaB phosphorylation, reduce NF-kappaB translocation to the nucleus to then transcribe inflammatory signaling, reduce the expression of COX-2, and reduce the enzyme inducible nitrogen oxide synthase [752].

---

750   Ng TB, Wang HX. Pharmacological actions of Cordyceps, a prized folk medicine. J Pharm Pharmacol. Dec 2005;57(12):1509-19.

751   Chiou YL, Lin CY. The extract of Cordyceps sinensis inhibited airway inflammation by blocking NF-kappaB activity. Inflammation. Jun 2012;35(3):985-93.

752   Ho GK et al. Cordycepin inhibits lipopolycaccharide-induced inflamamtion by the suppression of NF-kappaB through Akt and p38 inhibition in RAW 264.7 macrophage cells. European Journal of Pharmacology. 2006;545:192-199.

Dosing of Cordyceps is dictated by the purpose intended. Make sure the Cordyceps used is of the Cs-4 extract variety. General dosing is in the range of 200-400 mg daily. Even though no side effects have been reported, higher dosages of Cordyceps should occur under the care of a medical provider knowledgeable in the biochemical reactions of Cordyceps to maximize its effects and minimize any potential risks.

## Vitamin E

Vitamins E, like vitamin C is a powerful antioxidant. There are several different forms that make up the vitamin E family. There are the tocopherols (alpha, beta, gamma, and delta forms) and there is the tocotrienols (alpha, beta, gamma, and delta forms). That makes a total of 8 members of the vitamin E family [753] with the gamma tocopherol form as the most prevalent in the US diet and the alpha tocopherol form as the most dominant in the blood.

One aside. There was a recent firestorm over the proposed increased risk of prostate cancer with Vitamin E in the SELECT trial. What they failed to mention, was that the vitamin E used in this study (rac-alpha-tocopherol acetate) was a synthetic "inferior" form with well known toxic effects [754] [755]. Contrast that with other studies showing vitamin E's benefit in prostate disease [756] [757] [758] [759]. Studies have been mixed, but

---

753 Sen CK, Khanna S, Roy S. Tocotrienols: Vitamin E beyond Tocopherols. Life Sci. Mar 27 2006;78(18):2088-2098.

754 Chung YK, Mahan DC, Lepine AJ. Efficacy of dietary D-alpha tocopherol and DL-alpha-tocopheryl acetate for weanling pigs. J Anim Sci. Aug 1992;70(8):2485-92.

755 Diez Marques ML, Lucio Cazana FJ, Rodriguez Puyol M. In vitro response of erythrocytes to alpha-tocopherol exposure. Int J Vitam Nutr Res. 1986;56(3):311-5.

756 Weinstein SJ et al. Serum alpha-tocopherol and gamma-tocopherol in relation to prostate cancer risk in a prospective study. J Natl Cancer Inst. 2005;97(5):396-399.

757 Wada S. Chemoprevention of tocotrienols: the mechanism of antiproliferative effects. Forum Nutr. 2009;61:204-16.

758 Wada S et al. Tumor suppressive effects of tocotrienol in vivo and in vitro. Cancer Lett. Nov 18 2005;229(2):181-91.

759 Nesaretnam K. Multitargeted therapy of cancer by tocotrienols. Cancer Lett. Oct 8 2008;269(2):388-95.

it is clear that you should not use synthetic vitamin E. Natural vitamin E is ok and provides some degree of benefit in prostate health.

In addition to vitamin E's antioxidant properties, vitamin E helps to reduce inflammation. Alpha tocopherol, probably the most studied, has been shown to reduce CRP levels [760] and to reduce the inflammatory cytokine IL-1beta [761]. But, tocotrienols have been shown to provide greater CRP reduction compared to alpha tocopherols[762]. As a whole, vitamin E has been shown to inhibit NF-kappaB [763], induce apoptosis (programmed cell death), and recycle glutathione [764].

Of course, dietary intake of vitamin E is the best. As Vitamin E is a fat soluble vitamin, turn to fats for a good source of dietary Vitamin E. Good dietary sources of vitamin E include: nuts, seeds, egg yolks, olive oil, oatmeal, avocados, palm oil, rice bran, and green leafy vegetables. If oral supplementation is required, then dosing of vitamin E should include a mix of tocopherols and tocotrienols as the different forms of vitamin E have varied functions in the body [765]. I recommend an equal part of tocopherols and tocotrienols at 400 mg each daily. Vitamin E's are fat soluble and thus accumulate, so daily dosing may not be required for some.

---

760 Singh U, Devaraj S, Jialal I. Vitamin E, oxidative stress, and inflammation. Annu Rev Nutr. 2005;25:151-74.

761 Devaraj S, Jialal I. Alpha-tocopherol decreases interleukin-1 beta release from activated human monocytes by inhibition of 5-lipoxygenase. Arterioscler Throm Basc Biol. Apr 1999. 19(4):1125-33.

762 Prasad K. Tocotrienols and cardiovascular health. Curr Pharm Des. 2011;17(21):2147-54.

763 Glauert HP. Vitamin E and NF-kappaB activation: a review. Vitam Horm. 2007;76:135-53.

764 Calfee-Mason KG, Lee EY, Spear BT, Glauert HP. Role of the p50 subunit of NF-kappaB in vitamin E-induced changes in mice treated with the peroxisome proliferator, ciprofibrate. Food Chem Toxicol. Jun 2008;46(6):2062-73.

765 Colombo ML. An update on Vitamin E, tocopherol and tocotrienol-Perspectives. Molecules. 2010;15:2103-2113.

## Silymarin

Silymarin is the active component of Milk thistle. Silymarin is only found in the seed shell of the milk thistle plant. Milk thistle is a very common herb used to aid and protect the liver. Milk thistle has been used to treat a wide variety of liver disease, including alcoholic liver disease, viral hepatitis, and toxin-induced liver disease [766]. Additional benefits of silymarin are: antioxidant [767], inhibits lipid peroxidation [768], stimulates phase I detoxification [769], and recycles glutathione [770]

One reason for Milk thistle's liver benefits is due to the anti-inflammatory effects of Silymarin. Silymarin inhibits NF-kappaB activation [771], silymarin inhibits 5-lipoxygenase [772] [773], silymarin inhibits leukocyte migration to the site of inflammation [774], and silymarin inhibits IL-1B and prostaglandin E2 production [775]. Silymarin is a very active tool in the inhibition of inflammation.

766  Abenavoli L, Capasso R, Millic N, Capasso F. Milk thistle in liver diseases: past, present, future. Phytother Res. Oct 2010;24(10):1423-32.

767  Wagner H. Plant constituents with antihepatotoxic activity. In: Beal JL, Reinhard E eds. *Natural Products as Medicinal Agents*. Stuttgart: hippokrates-Verlag:1981.

768  Bosisio E et al. Effect of the flavanolignans of *Silybum marianum* L. on lipid peroxidation in rat liver microsomes and freshly isolated hepatocytes. Pharmacol Res. 1992;25:147-154.

769  Halim AB et al. Biochemical effect of antioxidants on lipids and liver function in experimentally-induced liver damage. Ann Clin Biochem. 1997;34:656-663.

770  Campos R et al. Silbin dihemisuccinate protects against glutathione depletion and lipid peroxidation induced by acetaminophen on rat liver. Planta Med. 1989;55:417-419.

771  Manna SK, Mukhopadhyay A, Nguyen TV, Aggarwal BB. Silymarin suprresses TNF-induced activation of NF-kappaB, c-Jun N-Terminal Kinase and apoptosis. J of Immunol. Dec 15 1999;163(12):6800-6809.

772  Gupta OP et al. Anti-inflammatory and anti-arthritic activities of silymarin acting through inhibition of 5-lipoxygenase. Phytomedicine. Mar 2000;7(1):21-4.

773  Fiebrich F, Koch H. Silymarin, an inhibitor of lipoxygenase. Experentia. 1979;35:150-152.

774  La Puerta RD, Martinez E, Bravo L, Ahumada MC. Effect of silymarin on different acute inflammation models and on leukocyte migration. Journal of Pharmacy and Pharmacology. Sept 1996;48(9):968-970

775  Kang JS et al. Protection against lipopolysaccharide-induced sepsis and inhibition of interleukin-1beta and prostaglandin E2 synthesis by silymarin. Biochemical

As milk thistle is of the daisy family, I don't expect anyone go out and eat Silybum marianum daily for their Silymarin. Instead, oral supplementation is the obvious choice. Silymarin is obtained through taking milk thistle as a standardized extract (79-80% silymarin). A good wellness dose is 300 mg twice daily. Dosing above that should be under the care of a medical provider familiar with Milk thistle.

## Coconut oil

Coconut has gotten a lot of publicity lately. Coconut oil has been promoted as great for dry skin and bulk for hair. Coconut is also a good fat to cook with. Coconut oil is a medium chain fatty acid that has been shown to have anti-inflammatory effects [776] [777]. Coconut oil has also been shown to reduce abdominal fat in 2 small studies [778] [779]. Just make sure it is Virgin coconut oil. These studies looked at 30 ml daily, which equates to 6 tsp daily–I hope you like your coconut!

## CoQ10

I encounter very few that have not heard of CoQ10. CoQ10 is a powerful antioxidant that is a part of the rate-limiting complex I of the electron transport chain (ETC). The ETC is the energy

---

Pharmacology. Jan 2004;67(1):175-181.

776  Intahphuak S, Khonsung P, Panthong A. Anti-inflammatory, analgesic, and anti-pyretic activities of virgin coconut oil. Pharm Biol. Feb 2010;48(2):151-7.

777  Zakaria ZA, Somchit MN, Mat Jais AM, Teh LK, Salleh MZ, Long K. In vivo anti-nociceptive and anti-inflammatory activities of dried and fermented processed virgin coconut oil. Med Princ Pract. 2011;20(3):231-6.

778  Assunacao ML Ferreira HS, dos Santos AF, Cabral CR Jr, Florencio TM. Effects of dietary coconut oil on the biochemical and anthropometric profiles of women presenting abdominal obesity. Lipids. Jul 2009;44(7):593-601.

779  Liau KM, Lee YY, Chen CK, Rasool AHG. An open-label pilot study to assess the efficacy and safety of virgin coconut oil in reducing visceral adiposity. ISRN Pharmacol. 2011;2011:949686.

pathway found in the mitochondria. Mitochondria are call the "power houses" of the cell because of this pathway and CoQ10 is the rate limiting complex in this pathway. Now you see why statin therapies can be so dangerous. Statins poison the CoQ10 dependent protein complex and compromise the energy production pathway–not good. That is the reason for the muscular pain associated with CoQ10. Low CoQ10 levels have been associated with many different chronic diseases of aging [780][781]. When you get down to it, the basics of life is can your cell make energy. If the cell doesn't have the ability to make energy it dies. When enough cells die, tissue dies, then organs, then the whole organism. The ability of the mitochondria to make energy is very important. Anything that disrupts that process is dangerous.

CoQ10 has been shown to aid cardiovascular disease [782][783][784], improve diabetes control [785], and aid in neurodegenerative disease [786][787]. As an antioxidant, CoQ10 does this through a reduction in inflammation.

780 Passi S, De PO, Puddu P, Littarru GP. Lipophillic antioxidants in human sebum and aging. Free Radic Res. Apr 2002;36(4):471-7.

781 Kontush A, Schippling S, Spranger T, Beisiegel U. Plasma ubiquinol-10 as a marker for disease: is the assay worthwhile? Biofactors. 1999;9(2-4):225-9.

782 Dhanasekaran M, Ren J. The emerging role of coenzyme Q-10 in aging, neurodegeneration, cardiovascular disease, cancer, and diabetes mellitus. Curr Neurovasc Res. Dec 2005;2(5):447-59.

783 Roseffeldt FL et al. Coenzyme Q10 protects the agin heart against stress: studies in rats, human tissues, and patients. Ann NY Acad Sci. Apr 2002;959:355-9.

784 Fotino AD, Thompson-Paul AM, Bazzano LA. Effect of coenzyme Q10 supplementation on heart failure: a meta-analysis. Am J Clin Nutr. Feb 2013;97(2):268-275.

785 Hodgson JM, Watts GF, Playford DA, Burke V, Croft KD. Coenzyme Q10 improves blood pressure and glycaemic control: a controlled trial in subjects with type 2 diabetes. Eur J Clin Nutr. Nov 2002;56(11):1137-42.

786 Somayajulu M et al. Role of mitochondria in neuronal cell death induced by oxidative stress;neuroprotection by Coenzyme Q10. Neurobiol Dis. Apr 2005;18(3):618-27.

787 Matthews RT, Yang L, Browne S, Baik M, Beal MF. Coenzyme Q10 administration increases brain mitochondrial concentrations and exerts neuroprotective effects. Proce Natl Acad Sci USA. Jul 21 1998;95(15):8892-7.

CoQ10 has been shown to reduce CRP (not just any CRP, but high sensitivity CRP) and IL-6 [788]. CoQ10 also reduces inflammatory signaling through NF-KappaB inhibition [789].

CoQ10 exists in two forms Ubiquinol and Ubiquinone. The difference between the two is that Ubiquinol is the reduced form and Ubiquinone is not. The reduced form of Ubiquinol is the active form of CoQ10. Taking the active form of a compound is always a better method of dosing. This way, one can achieve higher levels faster with lower dosing. Achieve the best with the least.

The optimal dosage of CoQ10 depends on the intended purpose. I always tell my clients that if they are over 40, they need to take 100 mg. Consider adding 100 mg for each successive decade. If you are on statin therapy, add in another 100 mg. You can see that I like CoQ10. Make sure it is the reduced, active form Ubiquinol.

I could go on and on. Some have more studies of support than others. There are many other therapies available to inhibit inflammation. Arginine, a common amino acid supplement, has been shown to reduce inflammation in animal [790] and in humans studies [791]. Allicin from garlic has been shown to reduce the pro-inflammatory cytokine TNF-alpha [792]. The soy isoflavone genistein has been

---

788  Lee BJ, Huang YC, Chen SJ, Lin PT. Effects of coenzyme Q10 supplementation on inflammatory markers (high-sensitivity C-reactive protein, interleukin-6, and homocysteine) in patients with coronary artery disease. Nutrition. Jul 2012;28(7-8):767-72.

789  Ebadi M, Sharma SK, Wanpen S, Amornpan A. Coenzyme Q10 inhibits mitochondrial complex-1 down-regulation and nuclear factor-kappa B activation. J Cell Mol Med. Apr-Jun 2004;8(2):213-22.

790  Hnia K et al. L-arginine decreases inflammation and modulates the nuclear factor-kappaB/matrix metalloproteinase cascade in mdx muscle fibers. Am J Pathol. Jun 2008;172(6):1509-19

791  Ingrid HC Vos et al. L-arginine supplementation improves function and reduces inflammation in renal allografts. JASN. Feb 1 2001;12(2):361-367.

792  Lang A et al. Allicin inhibits spontaneous and TNF-alpha induced secretion of proinflammatory cytokines and chemokines from intestinal epithelial cells. Clin

shown to reduce inflammation [793] [794]. We are all familiar with blue-berries and black berries, but bilberries, rich in polyphenols reduce inflammation [795]. Who doesn't love the herb ginger. Ginger has long been known to have great benefits in inflammation reduction [796]. The flavonoid apigenin found in many fruits, has been shown to inhibit TNF-alpha induced NF-kappaB activity [797]. Chinese skull cap, an herb, has been shown to reduce inflammation comparable to naproxen [798]. Cat's claw, an amazon vine, has been shown to inhibit inflammation through TNF-alpha inhibition [799].

As one can see, there are numerous ways to battle inflammation that don't involve drugs. Many natural anti-inflammatories can be found in the foods that we cook, the herbs that we use, and through the many supplements present over the counter.

The supplements and dosing described above should be taken under the care of a medical provider knowledgable in their benefits and side effects.

Nutr. Oct 2004;23(5):1199-208.

793  Vedrengh M, Jonsson IM, Holmdahl R, Tarkowski A. Genistein as an anti-inflammatory agent. Inflamm Res. Aug 2003;52(8):341-6.

794  Hua Lu et al. Genistein, a soybean isoflavone, reduces the production of pro-inflammatory and adhesion molecules induced by hemolysat in brain microvascular endothelial cells. 2009;109(1):32-37.

795  Kolehmainen M et al. Bilberries reduce low-grade inflammation in individuals with features of metabolic syndrome. Mol Nutr Food Res. Oct 2012;56(10):1501-10.

796  Grzanna R, Lindmark L, Frondoza CG. Ginger-an herbal medicinal product with broad anti-inflammatory actions. J Med Food. Summer 2005;8(2):125-32.

797  Funakoshi-Tago M, Nakamura K, Tago K, Mashino T, Kasahara T. Anti-inflammatory activity of structurally related flavonoids, Apigenin, Luteolin, and Fisetin. Int Immunopharmacol. Sep 2011;11(9):1150-9.

798  Levy RM et al. Flavocoxid is as effective as naproxen for managing the signs and symptoms of osteoarthritis of the knee in humans: a short-term randomized, double-blind pilot study. J Pediatr Gastroenterol Nutr. Dec 1985;4(6):923-30.

799  Hardin SR. Cat's claw: an Amzaonian vine decreases inflammation in osteoarthritis. Complement Ther Clin Pract. Feb 2007;13(1):25-8.